CTE, Media, and the NFL

Lexington Studies in Health Communication

Series Editor: Leandra H. Hernández and Kari Nixon

National and international governments have recognized the importance of widespread, timely, and effective health communication, as research shows that accurate, patient-centered, and culturally competent health communication can improve patient and community health care outcomes. This interdisciplinary series examines the role of health communication in society and is receptive to manuscripts and edited volumes that use a variety of theoretical, methodological, interdisciplinary, and intersectional approaches. We invite contributions on a variety of health communication topics including but not limited to health communication in a digital age; race, gender, ethnicity, class, physical abilities, and health communication; critical approaches to health communication; feminisms and health communication; LGBTQIA health; interpersonal health communication perspectives; rhetorical approaches to health communication; organizational approaches to health communication; health campaigns, media effects, and health communication; multicultural approaches to health communication; and international health communication. This series is open to contributions from scholars representing communication, women's and gender studies, public health, health education, discursive analyses of medical rhetoric, and other disciplines whose work interrogates and explores these topics. Successful proposals will be accessible to an interdisciplinary audience, advance our understanding of contemporary approaches to health communication, and enrich our conversations about the importance of health communication in today's health landscape.

Titles in the Series

CTE, Media, and the NFL: Framing a Public Health Crisis as a Football Epidemic, by Travis R. Bell, Janelle Applequist, and Christian Dotson-Pierson

Challenging Reproductive Control and Gendered Violence in the Americas: Intersectionality, Power, and Struggles for Rights, by Leandra Hinojosa Hernández and Sarah De Los Santos Upton

Politics, Propaganda, and Public Health: A Case Study in Health Communication and Public Trust, by Laura Crosswell and Lance Porter

Communication and Feminist Perspectives on Ovarian Cancer, by Dinah Tetteh

CTE, Media, and the NFL

Framing a Public Health Crisis as a Football Epidemic

Travis R. Bell, Janelle Applequist, and Christian Dotson-Pierson

LEXINGTON BOOKS
Lanham • Boulder • New York • London

Published by Lexington Books
An imprint of The Rowman & Littlefield Publishing Group, Inc.
4501 Forbes Boulevard, Suite 200, Lanham, Maryland 20706
www.rowman.com

6 Tinworth Street, London SE11 5AL

British Library Cataloguing in Publication Information Available

Library of Congress Cataloging-in-Publication Data Available

ISBN 978-1-4985-7056-5 (cloth)
ISBN 978-1-4985-7057-2 (electronic)
ISBN 978-1-4985-7058-9 (pbk.)

Contents

Preface

The idea for this book started in 2015, and the spark ignited on December 3, 2015. Janelle and I attended a speaking engagement at the Straz in downtown Tampa, Florida, to hear Dr. Bennet Omalu talk about the *Concussion* movie that would debut on Christmas Day. We jotted down pages of notes about Omalu, his fight with the National Football League over scientific findings, and this mysterious disease called chronic traumatic encephalopathy, or CTE as it was widely known at the time of his talk. CTE threatened the core of American sport—the NFL.

During this time, I was working on my Ph.D. in communication at the University of South Florida. The following spring semester in a health communication class, I wrote about how media framed CTE, Omalu, and the NFL related to the movie. Janelle helped code the news articles for the paper with a goal to submit to it to the National Communication Association (NCA) annual convention in November 2016. The paper titled "*Concussion*, Omalu, and the NFL: A quantitative analysis of a media template" was accepted. At NCA in Philadelphia, we met with Jimmy Hamill, an assistant acquisitions editor for Lexington Books. He had reached out to set up meeting to discuss the paper and the possibility to further develop this idea. Writing a book was never a thought until that meeting, and more than two years later, it happened.

Christian joined the project in 2017 after we reconnected following a brief introduction at NCA in 2015. Her interest in concussions and sports communication was a valuable addition to our research team. After several Skype meetings and phone calls, the book was underway with Lexington. We gathered news stories and started reading at length about this invisible disease, player deaths, and long-term memory loss. The stories were depressing, but the way media discussed it consistently made CTE a football problem. Thus, we had to find the truth.

Over twelve years of examining news stories, this book corroborated our intuition. CTE and the NFL joined an imperfect union fueled by scientists and journalists who wanted to better understand why prominent athletes were dying so young because they lost their mind, either over time or through sudden acts of violence. These events, along with misguided NFL medical research about concussions in football, forced the league to recognize this problem, albeit years after they should have. During this journey, media did some good things to raise public awareness of inherent risks, but in the process, excluded nearly every other sport and female athletes who can be at-risk because brain injuries show no sporting favoritism. Therefore, this book also hopes to raise awareness to anyone who should know about CTE. This includes athletes, parents, coaches, administrators, journalists, politicians, and other public figures.

We would like to acknowledge several people who helped make this book happen. First, the acquisition team at Lexington has been wonderful, beginning with Jimmy and then with Nicolette Amstutz and Jessica Tepper. I especially want to thank USF, who awarded a professional development leave for the fall 2017 semester to truly start this project. Professor Jen O'Brien is a friend and wonderful resource who helped us in the early stages of creating a code book to formulate a plan for our best research opportunity. Then in the spring 2018 semester, four student coders provided hours of their time to dive into the newspaper articles, help redevelop the code book, and dive deeper on second and third attempts to reach statistical reliability. Therefore, thank you to Kelsey Baker, Ifeoluwa Bolujo, Jasmine Burnett, and Ala Kader for your tireless effort to help make this book a success. Finally, we give a heartfelt thanks to the USF library staff who work on interlibrary loans. They helped find dozens of research articles and book chapters that provide significant context throughout the book. Finally, thank you to Janelle and Christian for helping guide this book project to be as inclusive and insightful as it could be. You are wonderful colleagues and friends.

This book is dedicated to the athletes who have lost their lives to CTE or any other brain disease as well as to the family members who have suffered as a result and are left to tell the story. We hope this book helps recognize that playing sports, not just football, put people at-risk of brain injury. Scientists have debated whether CTE is a real disease. Regardless if it should be described or named differently, the public understanding is that it is real, and it can be deadly. Therefore, we need to take the time to better define it, understand it, and educate about it so that parents can make a most-informed decision whether their child should start the risk.

ONE

Football and the Brain

A Historical Perspective

The National Football League (NFL) provides a spectacle unmatched by any sport in the United States (Oriard, 2014b), both in viewership and revenue. Despite a dip in television ratings in 2017 for the first time in decades, the NFL distributed $8.1 billion to its thirty-two franchises and added to the league's estimated $14 billion in overall revenue reported in 2017 (Carpenter, 2018). Most of this revenue was created through multimedia contracts and advertising income that reached $3.5 billion annually. The games and stadiums are filled with masculinity, nationalism, pageantry, and violence that feed an insatiable fan base and produce television ratings that networks pay billions to retain. In a culture that has built itself on encouraging violence and physical aggression, the NFL has been historically celebrated for its toughest, most injury-inducing hits that garner media attention and "reify hegemonic sporting masculinity as worthy" (Anderson & Kian, 2012, p. 156). Beyond a rabid fan base, the NFL is a global enterprise due in large part to its unique marketability fueled by a "cost-free athletic labor pool" (Meggyesy, 2000, p. 28) that receives its extensive professional training from colleges and universities before they ever reach the league.

However, a different spin on the religious experience of football was revealed with the 2015 theatrical release of *Concussion*. Despite problematic linguistic use of the term concussion in relation to a film about a doctor who had no connection to concussion diagnoses, the film served to bring the issue of brain injuries in football to a new public space of critique (Lau, 2016; Wilbur & Myers 2016). The film also helped to raise awareness of—and generate conversation around—chronic traumatic encephalopathy, or CTE as it is more commonly understood and discussed in mainstream dialogue. Thus, the film offered a new interpretation on a topic heavily discussed in the popular press that pressured media—along with football executives, coaches, players, parents, and doctors—to discuss CTE in a new light. This movie along with documentary films, books, long-form journalism, and medical research bound CTE into a lifelong relationship with the NFL.

Concussion built upon the work of multiple journalists who spent years uncovering a cause-and-effect result of brain injuries through contact sports, with American football as the exemplar. As Fainaru-Wada and Fainaru (2013) described in their thorough book, *League of Denial*, "there has never been anything like it in the history of sports: a public health crisis that emerged from the playing fields of our twenty-first century pastime. A small group of research scientists put football under a microscope—literally" (p. 6). The Fainaru brothers outlined how the NFL played a significant role in covering up the concern of brain injuries in football and attempted to discredit the science that worked to highlight this growing epidemic in America's favorite sport. In the process, doctors like Bennet Omalu and Ann McKee became household names and oppositional voices in media reports and congressional hearings to challenge the NFL and its hold on a public obsessed with American football (Laskas, 2009; Oaklander, Park, Durcharme, & Marty, 2018). In this process, the NFL reached a crossroads between on-field success and off-field credibility related to player safety directly connected to the brain. With the release of each new medical report and its coinciding media coverage, public opinion of the NFL continues to question the validity and the sanctity of the league and re-shape a national narrative in its representation of football from masculine autonomy to an increased awareness of the violent repercussions that result in contact sports However, this new awareness has not altered the league's success as evidenced by the continued ratings (albeit a slight dip) and revenue success.

As scientific research continued to increase the number of brains made available for examination and subsequent CTE diagnoses, media attention and focus centered on former athletes, especially players with NFL ties as if they were a sole participant in each study. For example, Mez et al. (2017) published a report in the *Journal of the American Medical Association* (JAMA) that examined 202 brains of deceased football players ranging in age from youth football players to those with years of NFL experience. The study found evidence of CTE in 177 (88%) of the donated brains. A subsequent survey of headlines from July 26, 2017, the day after the study was published, revealed a common theme centered squarely on NFL players.

> "C.T.E. is found in 110 of 111 donated N.F.L. brains."
>
> —*The New York Times*

> "Out of 111 former NFL players, only one didn't have CTE."

—*The Mercury News*

"Study finds CTE in 99% of ex-NFL brains."

—*The Washington Post*

"BRAIN PAIN: In new study of ex-NFL players, 99 percent had CTE."

—*New York Daily News*

The fact that media outlets extensively focused on the NFL was not surprising given the league's popularity in American society. What should be recognized is that the remaining 91 brains, of which 67 (74%) exhibited CTE, received minimal recognition in news headlines, which often act to provide the "hook" to entice someone to read a full story.

This one moment in time produced two mediated thoughts for audiences if the stories were never read beyond their headlines. First, if someone plays in the NFL, they will get CTE. Second, CTE is almost exclusively a football problem. Fundamentally, this provides a snapshot of how media frame issues within their reporting and how media framing functions, whereby media select what to include in the limited space afforded to newspapers and the frequency in which individuals or groups are associated with a given story. Thus, media construct understanding for readers through a process of selection, salience, and omission (Entman, 1993; Gitlin, 1980). This process of media framing is the foundation of this book. Yes, CTE is pervasive in football and across many other contact sports as this book identifies. However, media discourse through ideological journalistic practices has framed CTE in a relationship with the NFL dating to 2005 when the brains of football player Mike Webster and neuropathologist Bennet Omalu became inextricably linked (Alosco, Healy, & Stern, 2019), which is outlined in chapter 3. Regardless of what information new studies reveal about the prevalence of CTE in other sports, media attention remains on American football and overwhelmingly frames CTE within the context of the NFL. Therefore, CTE and the NFL serve as parallel acronyms of the violent outcome of playing America's most popular sport.

The scope of this book is to examine the mediated construction of CTE and its rise to public and political prominence by way of its direct connection with the NFL. More broadly, this book explores how this relationship situates in and through a sports/media complex (Jhally, 1984; Jhally, 1989) created via television, fueled by other forms of mass media, and blurred between major international media conglomerates and the world's most influential sports league. To achieve this correlation, the book serves to achieve several goals: (1) trace how newspapers framed CTE and what role media play in constructing CTE broadly as a football problem, and more specifically an issue almost exclusive to the NFL; (2) examine how film interpreted this mediated narrative to present CTE through popular culture; (3) examine how these mediated storylines disrupt the long-standing intersection of masculinity and football; and (4) analyze how constructing a CTE/NFL relationship influences and indirectly impacts other sports that face issues of brain injuries as well as implications moving forward into political and societal spaces.

Before outlining the chapters in this book, two brief overview sections provide a foundation for what this book examines within media framing, which is the theoretical guide explained extensively in chapter 2. First, a synopsis of American football and its connection to violence, masculinity, and brain injuries offers historical context for the status of the game in relation to player safety and head injuries. Second, definitions for and differentiations between concussion and CTE provide a basic framework to understand medical terminology that drives this research.

FOOTBALL AND BRAIN INJURIES

The most commonly referenced first football game was played between Princeton and Rutgers in 1869, but it has been contested for its connection to modern American football since it was described as "a college soccer football game" ("Chronology of," 2017) that used modified soccer rules. The current form of football was attributed to a college game played in 1874 between McGill and Harvard that more closely resembled rugby (Guttmann, 2006). What has been consistently agreed upon was that American football as a "*collision* sport" (Oriard, 2014a, p. 126) produced a naturalized environment of violence. This concern since the sport's inception was quickly raised when annual player deaths consistently reached double digits, primarily the result of faulty (or no) equipment and minimal regulatory oversight on the field (Dunn, Dunn, & Day, 2006). American football produced the greatest number of head injuries in sport and resulted in eighteen deaths in college football in 1905 (Zezima, 2014). That same year, President Theodore Roosevelt gathered coaches and athletic directors from Ivy League schools in a meeting that *The Washington Post* reported would "start the ball rolling in the direction of a modification of the rules of the game" ("Hears football men," 1905). Roosevelt's motives to get involved have been questioned because despite numerous rule changes that followed, the number of deaths continued by the dozens with a peak of thirty-one in 1931 (Oriard, 2014a) and with minimal acceptance of the risk of head injuries among the participants.

In a study monitoring the injuries of the 1905 Harvard football team, head injuries were regarded with little consequence. Nichols and Smith (1906) noted that a "concussion was treated by the players in general as a trivial injury and rather regarded as a joke" (p. 3). The authors did not regard concussions as lightly and added that after speaking with neurologists there was "the possibility of serious after effects" (p. 3) from repetitive physical contact that produced frequent concussions both in practice and games. Additionally, it was reported that only two games during that season did not produce at least one concussion and that surgeons on the sidelines were often first to recognize a player suffering from a head injury because "a player might, apparently, automatically run through a considerable series of plays before his mates noticed that he was mentally irresponsible" (p. 3). Lastly of importance from this study, memory loss was noted to range from a few minutes to a week and that players must be examined immediately to avoid the possibility of brain hemorrhage. These findings and recommendations sound eerily like those throughout the twenty-first century, which indicates the longevity of awareness of potential brain injuries specific to American football but with challenging advances in diagnosis and treatment.

This lack of adherence to or concern for risks associated with football illuminates the gendered socializing force of masculinity. Sabo and Gordon (1995) attributed this socialization process to when "boys adopt masculine behaviors, which, in turn, can impact their susceptibility to illness or accidental deaths" (p. 6). The foundational intersection of masculinity and sport, according to Messner (1990), "emerged as a male response to social changes which undermined many of the bases of men's traditional patriarchal power, authority, and identity" (p. 204). American football ideally situated as a uniquely male space that worked to preclude women through constructing a sport that was inherently masculine and aggressive (McDowell & Schaffner, 2011). Thus, football served as a socializing agent to assert violence with minimal regard to risk, which ultimately served as a proving ground for men to be tough and fight through pain (Sabo, 2009). This was clear in the study of the 1905 Harvard football team. Additionally, media historically played a role in compromising health risks in contact sports by defending and highlighting the violence (Young, White, & McTeer, 1994).

Despite an understanding that football was a physical endeavor with inherent health risks, college football grew in popularity, in large part through a symbiotic relationship with media (Montez de Oca, 2013). Organized professional football would follow in 1920 with the formation of the American Professional Football Conference. The conference was renamed the National Football League on June 24, 1922 ("Chronology of," 2017). Both college and professional football evolved through rule changes and equipment modifications aimed at making the sport safer to combat the rising number of player deaths, but these adaptations focused on fatalities and failed to consider the concern for head injuries (Harrison, 2014). Plastic helmets replaced the original leather versions in 1939 with a targeted goal of reducing skull fractures. Face masks were added in 1956. These changes trickled down to the high school level that witnessed a significant decrease in head and neck injuries (Alley, 1964). These technological advancements may have reduced the total number of reported head injuries, but these advances have been questioned as a cause for concern in football where the newly developed equipment provides a sense of invincibility and offers potential for use as a weapon instead of protection (Anderson & Kian, 2012).

The concern over football fatalities spawned a survey started in 1931 by the American Football Coaches Association to track the number and cause of fatalities directly and indirectly related to football. The records are updated annually by the National Center for Catastrophic Sport Injury Research at the University of North Carolina at Chapel Hill. Between 1931 and 2016, the survey identified 1,848 fatalities in football across all levels with 1,048 as a direct result of football. The report is divided into four categories: (1) organized youth, (2) middle and high school, (3) college, and (4) professional and semi-pro. Middle and high school football players account for nearly two-thirds (n = 696, 66.4%) of direct football fatalities, followed by organized youth (n = 179, 17.1 percent), college (n = 92, 8.8 percent), and professional/semi-pro (n = 81, 7.7 percent). This split is not surprising considering that roughly 3,000,000 youth participate in football while 1.1 million high schoolers play the sport. Clearly the physicality of high school players versus young children would place a significant impact on the greater number of deaths along with modified rules for youth football. In comparison, approximately 100,000 football players compete beyond the high school level combined across all collegiate associations, semi pro, and professional, with approximately 1,500 players on NFL rosters during any given season (Kucera, Klossner, Colgate, & Cantu, 2017). Regardless of proportion, the number of deaths is alarming and a result of the environmental risk and hazard of playing football.

A noticeable decrease in the number of deaths occurred in 1976 following a rule change aimed at eliminating leading with the head and face both for blocking and tackling that was attributed to the findings of this annual survey. The National Collegiate Athletic Association (NCAA) in 1978 and the National Federation of State High School Associations (NFHS) in 1980 adopted helmet technical standards established by the National Operating Committee on Standards for Athletic Equipment (NOCSAE). These changes had a direct effect on a decrease in football fatalities with a banner (and only) year in 1990 without a direct football-related death. Of importance to this book, most of the direct fatalities since 1960 were caused by brain and neck injuries. Even more alarming, since the 1990 anomaly, 72 of the 120 deaths (60 percent) were a direct result of a brain injury (Kucera et al, 2017).

Each story of a player's death on the football field now receives media attention, and rightfully so. However, without a death during an NFL game as a direct result of the sport, these stories are considered isolated events that often quickly fade beyond a short media shelf life and are attributed to a range of causes. Only one player has ever died during an NFL game. In 1971, Chuck Hughes suffered a heart attack while playing wide receiver for the Detroit Lions. It was later discovered that the twenty-eight-year-old had an undiagnosed family history of a heart condition (Maron, 2015). The NFL was less than two years removed from a merger with the competing American Football League and had only completed five Super Bowl games. The league was rapidly growing in popularity, but limited media attention centered on Hughes unlike if his unfortunate death had occurred in the media-infused era of the 2000s that is obsessed with American football.

The NFL has implemented countless rule changes in hopes of avoiding anyone dying on the field. The league could be heralded for championing a cause for player safety, but a counter argument could be that the league is only concerned with player safety while they are active players who generate revenue for the league. After a player completes his career, he produces little economic benefit for the league and is left with a lifetime of lasting injuries. While bodily injuries are visible evidence of the physical toll of playing football, brain injuries are the ones invisible to fans, television cameras, and even doctors. However, it is these invisible injuries and long-term effects that threaten the NFL's success and popularity. Linked as an indirect cause in several highly publicized player deaths like Mike Webster, Junior Seau, and Dave Duerson (Korngold, Farrell, & Fozdar, 2013), brain injuries and the medically rejuvenated CTE provide a charged topic consistently connected to the NFL that requires greater understanding and provides a potential threat to football that for decades was "culturally equated" (Sabo & Jansen, 1992, p. 169) with masculinity through an omnipresent construction and collection of glorified media imagery. The NFL's history of research surrounding brain injuries that attempted to deflect media attention to these risks is explored throughout this book, but first some clarification is necessary between the two most commonly discussed terms connected to brain injuries in sport.

CONCUSSION VS. CTE

Concussion and CTE are often invariably linked, but there are distinctions between these two brain injuries, which are blurred in published research and media reports (Asken & Bauer, 2018). At a basic level, CTE has a pathological meaning, and concussion does not (Sharp & Jenkins, 2015). However, it is important to borrow from the head injury literature and establish a baseline for attempting to understand the problem at hand despite a lack of clarity for how to assess the issue (Randolph, 2011).

First and foremost, concussion is a popular term but simply is a sport-specific reference for a mild traumatic brain injury (mTBI), which is the most frequent type of traumatic brain injury (TBI). The Glasgow Coma Scale was established in 1974 to determine severity of head injuries. The test examines functionality and responsiveness, then categorizes the injury as either mild (mTBI), moderate (MTBI), or severe based on a patient's eye opening, verbal response, and motor response (Teasdale & Jennett, 1974; Teasdale et al., 2014). TBIs are classified by three mechanisms of cause: closed or blunt force, blast injury, or penetrating injury (O'Phelan, 2016). Athletes can be diagnosed with a sports-related concussion if they suffer some form of closed or blunt trauma to the head while in competition or practice, and concussions most often occur in contact with another athlete. Conversely, civilian and military diagnoses of similar injuries are discussed as mTBI. The brain injury is the same regarding cause and diagnosed severity. It is simply a linguistic difference for sport.

The Center for Disease Control and Prevention (CDC) tracks the frequency and type of TBIs in the United States. The CDC defines a TBI as "a bump, blow, or jolt to the head that disrupts the normal function of the brain" and identifies children and older adults as greater risks for TBI. In 2013, approximately 2.8 million people suffered a TBI that resulted in an emergency room visit, hospitalization, or death. Over a six-year span from 2007 to 2013, hospitalization increased 47 percent for TBI-related emergency room visits. Among children ages nineteen or younger, TBI diagnosis caused by sport- or recreation-related injuries reached nearly 330,000 in 2012, which was more than double the number reported in 2001 ("TBI: Get the facts," n.d.). The CDC launched a "Heads Up" campaign in 2003 focused on concussion prevention, recognition, and response among health care providers and expanded the program to sports partners aimed at sharing the information via microsites on organization websites as well as for parents and coaches through the CDC website for basics about brain injuries, proper helmet safety, and legal guidelines by state or organizational policies ("Heads Up," n.d.).

While concussion research and awareness into the early 2000s were medically documented and discussed in media, CTE research and public information was in its infancy and nearly non-existent. This paralleled a similar lack of clarity for understanding mTBI before the Glasgow Coma Scale was developed, introduced, and widely accepted as a diagnostic standard (Teasdale et al., 2014). As outlined, concussions are induced by some type of trauma that produces a *disturbance of brain function* but does not always result in a structural injury to the brain (Nowinski, 2007; O'Phelan, 2016). Where CTE differs from a concussion is in the *long-term structural effect* on the brain. These structural abnormalities result from brain trauma that diminishes brain volume. Brain trauma is required for a CTE diagnosis, and the neurodegenerative disease occurs with greater frequency in cases of *repeated* brain trauma over time (Montenigro et al., 2016a). However, CTE goes beyond sport to include abuse victims and military service members (Concannon, Kaufman, & Herring, 2014). Therefore, an important difference between concussion and CTE is through the repetitive occurrence of brain trauma that produces structural damage over time to the brain beyond a single blow that disturbs brain function.

This idea of repetitive brain trauma resulting in CTE was not new in the medical community (Corsellis, Bruton, & Freeman-Browne, 1973; Critchley 1949, 1957; Johnson, 1969), but it was primarily limited to boxing, which is outlined in the historical evolution of CTE in chapter 4. CTE advanced beyond medical journals and entered the public sphere once an American football player was diagnosed with the disease (Omalu et al., 2005). Since then, awareness and coverage have reached captivating levels from sports-governing bodies, legal and congressional intervention, and a slew of medical researchers garnering significant headlines with each new case study despite the disease not being recognized as an official cause of death (Lehman, Hein, Baron, & Gersic, 2012). There are many debates regarding diagnosis, who is at risk, and symptoms unique to CTE compared to other neurodegenerative conditions. A growing concern among some medical professionals has been connected with how a limited scope of case studies produced what they contended as speculative data that resulted in a cascade of mediated information (Granier, Mcnamee, Cifu, & Goldberg, 2011; Iverson, 2016; Randolph, 2014).

No perfect or immediate diagnostic test exists for CTE, and a complete diagnosis is only available postmortem, which does not help in the immediate impact of living with CTE (Concannon et al., 2014; Montenigro, Sisniega, & Cantu, 2016b; Saffary, Chin, & Cantu, 2012). Outward physical symptoms, changes in mood, noticeable depression, and violence (either self-inflicted or to others) are discussed as potential signs of CTE, but the inability for imaging tests has further fueled mediated and clinical debates about long-term risks of head injuries and their connection to and/or cause of CTE. For example, multiple suicide deaths of former athletes were reported where they specifically avoided shooting themselves in the head to donate their brains for the study of CTE. Media reports continued to link CTE with depression and suicide, yet Iverson (2016) found NFL players to be at a lower risk for suicide than men in the general population and raised a concern that oversaturation of media stories linking CTE and suicide could heighten suicidal behavior in at-risk athletes.

A common misperception is that concussions cause CTE, which has often been inferred through media. Concussions can be a causal effect in CTE but are not always recognized in CTE diagnoses. Stein, Alvarez, and McKee (2015) reported that 16 percent of published CTE cases did not indicate a known history of concussions. Additionally, not all concussions result in CTE nor are there any required number of concussions that lead to CTE (Montenigro, Sisniega, & Cantu, 2016a). The overall sentiment is that brain injuries have been—and will continue to be—a concern in long-term cognitive impact connected to contact sports but that information and understanding that fuel discussion around potentially deadly consequences must be clarified.

The constant circulation of misinformation led to a need for some consistent measures for CTE, especially since symptoms are representative of several other diseases (e.g., Alzheimer's, Parkinson's) and inconsistent standards were not universally accepted based on differing pathological classifications (Gardner, Iverson, & McCrory, 2014; Hornbeck, Walter, & Myrvik, 2017). These diseases are often identified through a collection or clustering of tau that appear in different regions of the brain and are distinguished by pathological characteristics (McKee et al., 2009). A group of researchers gathered in 2015 to examine twenty-five cases of varying tauopathies to determine consensus neuropathological criteria to differentiate and diagnose CTE from other neurodegenerative conditions. The article was published by sixteen authors in *Acta Neuropathologica* and determined that "the p-tau pathology of CTE is clearly distinct from other tauopathies" (McKee et al., 2016, p. 80) but also noted that additional research must help "determine the nature and degree of brain injury necessary to cause this neurodegeneration" (p. 82). Therefore, consensus criteria were established pathologically but little was added for causation beyond repeated exposure to brain trauma that had been established over the past seventy years of research that suggested "a clear environmental origin" (Love & Solomon, 2014, p. 1261) for CTE rooted in contact sports with a connection between head injuries and neuropathological changes.

As research on brain injuries and CTE continued to evolve, a second issue beyond diagnostic limitations quickly followed as an availability cascade, specifically related to risk, bias, and public perception. Kuran and Sunstein (1999) explain that availability cascades are generated by various social mechanisms, including media and policymakers, where "expressed perceptions trigger chains of individual responses that make these perceptions appear increasingly plausible through their rising availability in public discourse" (p. 685). Rapid circulation of information can produce availability errors and lead to "mass delusions" (p. 685) caused by limited, but explosive, cases fueled by intense media coverage that effects laws and policies despite availability errors. Kuran and Sunstein outline three such cases: (1) chemical waste dumping in the Love Canal in upstate New York, (2) pesticides in fruits that cause tumors, and (3) regulatory changes in the wake of the TWA flight 800 crash. In each case, oversaturation of media coverage influenced public perception and policy. The authors identify that availability cascades are not new but that they "can arise with respect to any issue on which large numbers of people have limited knowledge" (p. 763) that can have long-term social effects.

Availability cascades can apply to any topic, but public health concerns fit the protocol quite nicely in that they can generate media storms centered on surges of information (Vasterman, 2018). Specific to medical research, bias is a significant concern that can produce availability cascade examples. Medical research prefers randomized controlled trials (RCT) to avoid selection bias that can skew data and provide fuel for public outcry. Two types of biases can influence selection bias. First, ascertainment bias "occurs when the results or conclusions of a trial are systematically distorted by knowledge of which intervention each participant is receiving" (Jadad & Enkin, 2007, p. 33) and the best way to avoid this bias is to hide identities. Second, sampling bias is of significant concern for inclusion or exclusion of patients for research but is difficult to avoid in specific categories of research, including brain injuries, because it is difficult to randomize a sample of brain injuries since they are often caused by an external, sometimes accidental, factor. Lack of control groups mixed with potentially biased samples is where the concern over CTE is raised and its resulting availability cascade.

The availability cascade for CTE is especially perplexing because a control group is virtually impossible since postmortem diagnosis is the only option and brains must be donated (Alosco et al., 2019), which are often provided by family members because of expected conditions related to symptoms generated by the neurodegenerative disease that are widely circulated by media. Additionally, symptoms for CTE often do not appear until one or two decades after an athlete played her or his final game (Love & Solomon, 2014), which further clouds how to identify people for a possible sample to examine while they are living. With such a unique population at-risk for CTE, skewed data should be expected and was later quantified by Finkel and Bienick (2018) to explain that concerns surrounding a need for empirically and medically verifiable data should be overshadowed by a plausibly inherent risk between American football and CTE. During the rise of CTE in media discourse, the traction generated when a new study linking CTE and the NFL was released provided a pause to question data and only publish the eye-catching headlines. This creates a mediated societal problem at an intersection of media, medicine, and sport that is trapped between media performing its journalistic duty to inform the public about potential health concerns and medical researchers trying to highlight risks associated with a sport that carries social and cultural significance in American society.

WHAT'S AHEAD

This book is organized in three sections. The first section (chapters 2, 3, and 4) provides significant historical context to understand why and how this book examines the relationship between CTE and the NFL. The second section (chapters 5, 6, and 7) offers the media analysis, including twelve years of newspaper coverage and three important films in popular culture. The final section (chapters 8 and 9) outlines the impact of media framing on public understanding of CTE, missed opportunities that could help better contextualize brain injuries in sport, and the future of CTE in media.

Chapter 2 is critical to understand how media framing works by examining two cases studies of global epidemics that are central to the intersection of CTE and the NFL via the media lens. Media framing of the HIV/AIDS crisis in the 1980s and media representation of Big Tobacco throughout the twentieth century offer a background for how media would frame the NFL in relation to CTE during its rise to public prominence. Chapter 3 discusses the foundation of football as embedded in the American ideological perspective of hegemonic masculinity. Additionally, the influence of violence and war analogies in the NFL provide context for a culture less willing to accept brain injuries. Chapter 4 provides historical context for chronic traumatic encephalopathy by tracing its medical lineage from punch-drunk syndrome to dementia pugilistica to the reinvigorated status as CTE. Mike Webster and Bennet Omalu are presented in a contextualized relationship that started the mediated rise of CTE as an availability cascade in the NFL.

Chapters 5 and 6 provide a mixed methods analysis of 737 newspapers stories written between 2006 and 2017. This examination of six newspapers traces the role of journalism in constructing CTE as a public health crisis and a football epidemic. These two chapters offer historical perspective of how newspapers present information from headline-to-lead-to-text to synthesize how the mediated story of CTE unfolds. Chapter 7 examines three films connected to CTE in sport. This film critique explains the role of film as a form of slow journalism to delve into the stories embedded in the narrative intersection of CTE and the NFL.

Chapter 8 outlines two groups who were excluded from the mediated rise of CTE to public prominence. First, the omission of female athletes from the media narrative of brain injuries in sport runs contrary to scientific findings and reifies the masculine hold of American sport. Second, a myriad of other at-risk sports for brain injuries are identified beyond their tangential, and often minimal, inclusion in the mixed methods study for this book. Chapter 9 contextualizes the relationship between CTE and the NFL as a social phenomenon and availability cascade perpetuated by media. This chapter also forecasts where the CTE narrative might shift following the NFL's admission of a link to the disease in 2016. The authors hope this book provides a perspective of cultural, historical, and social significance in the recognition and risk of brain injuries in sport.

TWO

Framing Global Epidemics

A Case Study of HIV/AIDS and Big Tobacco

Media consumption in the United States means much more now than in past decades. In an ever-expanding arena of communication tools available at any given time, consumers have an ability to engage with multiple platforms of information. On a typical day, it is not uncommon for individuals to check their e-mail, browse various Internet sites, watch cable television, stream an Internet-based program, tune into the evening broadcast news, listen to the radio, catch a glimpse of headlines plastered on magazines in the grocery store's checkout line, and the list goes on. Media play a pivotal role in daily life. Beyond providing the foundation necessary to make daily decisions (e.g., weather, news, and entertainment), these forums also provide countless opportunities to engage in social learning. That is, media create and perpetuate various norms that reposition its role as a powerful socializing agent (Croteau & Hoynes, 1997; Kline, 2003).

MEDIA FRAMING OF HEALTH ISSUES

When addressing the topic of health, consideration of media's role in shaping public understanding cannot be underestimated. Media provide ubiquitous forums to derive knowledge regarding health risks to avoid, appropriate wellness measures to ensure a healthy lifestyle, and even epidemics on global scales that require immediate attention from various stakeholders (Hernández & de los Santos Upton, 2018). Media framing is an important issue to consider when discussing media's influence on health topics, including CTE. The ways in which the media report on lesser known health issues ultimately shapes how these topics will be socially constructed and subsequently understood. As such, this chapter seeks to define and explicate framing theory and its importance in the CTE conversation by providing two case studies showing framing's influence of previous health issues.

Framing theory states that media strategically frame issues in ways that lead the public to think in particular ways (Andsager & Powers, 1999; Andsager & Powers, 2001; Entman, 1991; Entman, 1993). Frames provide audiences with meaningful ways of looking at specific topics or issues, meaning that certain viewpoints become more legitimized, subsequently pushing other viewpoints out of the conversation (Entman, 1991; Jung, 2013; Parrott, 1996). Additionally, framing theory allows examination of individual news stories over time to understand how media construct them together into meaningful, centralized events (Gamson & Modigliani, 1987; Goffman, 1974; Tuchman, 1976). Studies such as the one in this book find media framing especially helpful when unpacking rapidly developing stories centered on health risks (e.g., CTE) as well as questioning powerful social institutions (e.g., NFL).

In discussing how public perception develops for a topic that reaches availability cascade levels, Kuran and Sunstein (1999) raise awareness for how biases and heuristics influence cognitive processes related to a cascading topic.

> A number of experiments have identified systematic problems in the ways people receive, store, retrieve, and process information. A particularly relevant problem stems from the *framing effect,* whereby given data are evaluated differently depending on how they are framed. A striking example is that people are more eager to undergo treatment for an ailment when they hear that ninety percent of patients treated five years ago are still alive than when they learn that ten percent of the treated patients have died. (p. 705)

This provides an interesting anecdote for framing, in which the same information presented two ways directly influenced who received the information simply by how it was presented. Kuran and Sunstein identify availability entrepreneurs who assist in framing what information is received and processed. In the case of CTE, availability entrepreneurs include athletes, the NFL and other sports governing bodies, medical professionals, lawyers, family members, and journalists. The centralizing agent and trigger for all entrepreneurs is media, which serve how, when, and what information circulates as well as why and to whom that information receives merit for dissemination.

This circular and intersectional overlap between availability entrepreneurs provides an example for how media framing works within two primary frames: media frames and individual frames (Scheufele, 1999). Media frames organize a story to filter information to a broader public for understanding of "what the controversy is about, the essence of the story" (Gamson & Modigliani, 1987, p. 143). Individual frames influence how that information is processed and synthesized through "short-term, issue-related frames of reference" (Scheufele, 1999, p. 107) that can include prior knowledge, direct connection to an issue or topic, interest in the story, or just a general desire to learn. Within that communication pattern of media sharing relevant and timely information, framing occurs through the *selection* of stories to report about and the *salience* of coverage that makes a story more prominent (Entman, 1993). How much information is shared or omitted and how often offer a method for media to organize discourse around an issue (Gitlin, 1980) that has shown throughout history to impact public perception regardless of whether the discussion centers on politics, medicine, public safety, war, or sports, just to name a few major topics. However, how media frame stories has shifted significantly over time with changing technologies available to share information more rapidly than ever before.

Media framing is considered one of three overarching media effects along with agenda-setting and priming. Each effect provides a different capacity that media play in shaping public knowledge and all three provide specific, but often overlapping, roles in the mediated process. Despite shifting trends of what defines media in the information age guided by online and social media, the concept of media framing still centers on shaping how stories are constructed. Thus, media, primarily in the traditional mass-mediated form, set an agenda for given issues and influence public perception through their salient coverage (McCombs & Shaw, 1972). Media frames of an issue are offered through packaged content that allow for a "degree of controversy" (Gamson & Modigliani, 1989, p. 3) dependent on who provides the information. Thus, an agenda is fluid depending on the evolution of a story that is guided by how stories are framed. After media frame an agenda, viewers and readers are primed to consider certain aspects of life while ignoring other information to render choices and judgements on the issue in question (Iyengar & Kinder, 1987). Through this process, varying levels of availability entrepreneurs enter and exit the conversation and help shape and re-shape public perception including government intervention, differing media organizations, and interest groups both for and against a given issue (Cohen, 1963). Therefore, all influential players in media and public discourse work together to shape a social construction of reality based on personal, interpersonal, and mediated interaction (Neuman, Just, & Crigler, 1992).

How and what media cover and the ways in which they frame health and safety risks has long been established as an important area for research (McCombs, 2004; Schiavo, 2007; Viswanath & Emmons, 2006). Multiple studies have shown that perceptions of health risks are associated with the extent of news coverage of those risks (Combs & Slovic, 1979;

Higgins, Naylor, Berry, O'Connor, & McLean, 2006; Lichtenstein, Slovic, Fischoff, Layman, & Combs, 1978). Beyond this, it has been found that news coverage of health matters can influence public policy and individual behavior (Yanovitzky & Bennett, 1999; Yanovitzsky, 2002). Therefore, given the large influence that media coverage can have on public health issues and attitudes, it becomes critical that research continue to understand the nature of coverage for various risks (Slater, Long, Bettinghaus, & Reineke, 2008).

Media influence health in two important ways. First, media may influence individual health behaviors whether such actions are for better or worse (Walsh-Childers, 2017). An example of this would be the ways in which advertising has normalized the existence of certain junk foods, potentially contributing to obesity in the United States. Another example would be considering how newspaper headlines discussing the Zika virus served as a form of important education for individuals previously unaware of the health crisis. Second, media have an ability to more indirectly influence social or physical environments by normalizing specific values (Walsh-Childers, 2017). In this sense, the ways media discuss health policy, legislative reform of health issues, or even the availability of health curricula in public schools each serve as ways media play a large role in our understanding of health. As described by Brown and Walsh-Childers (1994), there are, of course, multiple effects possible when considering media's role in health. Table 2.1 shows how media serve as a mediator for normalizing certain health behaviors and understandings, thus creating intended and unintended consequences that are important to consider.

To better show the ways in which media serve as an integral part in shaping society's understanding of important health topics, this chapter provides two case studies as exemplars of health phenomenon shaped largely by media discourse. The first case study examines how media framed the HIV/AIDS epidemic in context as an availability cascade. The second case study examines the intersection of media and the tobacco industry to unpack how relationships between media and major corporations can be problematic, especially when media is a vehicle to promote an industry that produces environmental risks. Note that the authors recognize the risk and deadly outcome of CTE is not comparable to HIV/AIDS, which still claims thousands of lives every year ("Global statistics," n.d.). Instead, the authors want to outline how media reports on science as it unfolds in real time without the assistance of longitudinal medical studies. It is important to note that Western interpretations of major health crises were chosen, and their subsequent media responses emphasized, as this book focuses on the influence of media on health in the United States. Also important to these two case studies was how they connected to dominant masculine ideology embedded in American culture, relevant to the consideration of the media's framing of CTE.

Table 2.1. *The Media Health Effects Matrix*

		Individual Behavior	Public Policy
Intended Effects	**Positive**	Traditional mass media campaigns; drug prevention programs;	Media advocacy campaigns; social campaigns supporting health policy improvements
	Negative	Tobacco advertising	Lobbying efforts coordinated in public campaigns to block anti-smoking efforts
Unintended Effects	**Positive**	Increased risk awareness; news coverage of health diagnoses; social media conversations about flu prevention	News agenda-setting or framing supports restrictions on alcohol advertising during daytime programming
	Negative	Increased "screen time" displaces exercise	News framing of the economic costs of environmental protection or the economic benefits of "fracking" discourage government investment in solar and wind technologies

Note: Adapted from Brown, J., & Walsh-Childers, K. (1994). *Effects of media on personal and public health*. In J. Bryant & D. Zillmann (Eds.), *Media effects: Advances in theory and research* (1st ed., pp. 389–415). Hillsdale, NJ: Lawrence Erlbaum Associates.

HIV/AIDS AND MORAL PANIC

AIDS continues to be a worldwide epidemic, contrary to a diminishing number of media reports (Cohen & You, 2018). The panic surrounding the outbreak of the HIV virus and subsequent disease known as AIDS largely stemmed from the media's erratic coverage of the epidemic (Dearing & Rogers, 1992; Swain, 2005). Approximately 72 percent of Americans reported receiving their information on AIDS directly from the media, pointing to the importance the media have in shaping the understanding of public health issues (Brodie, Hamel, Brady, Kates, & Altman, 2004; Watney, 1987). However, as Jonsen, Cooke, & Koenig (1986) interpreted in how media covered the AIDS epidemic,

> the turmoil of emotion stirred by the horror of the disease, its menace to the health of society, and its association with sexuality make almost impossible a dispassionate analysis that sorts out principle from prejudice and basic values from expedient policies. (p. 64)

In looking back on media's role in informing various publics, the initial confusion surrounding the progression of HIV and subsequent diagnoses of AIDS was interpreted as mediated panic, thus fueling further public confusion and misinformation being spread (Krishnan, Durrah, & Winkler, 1997; Labra, 2015).

Weeks (1989) was pivotal in acknowledging three definitive stages that occurred in shaping social representations of HIV/AIDS. The first stage (1981–1982), referred to as the "dawning crisis," was the point at which American media first began reporting on AIDS as associated with the four H's (heroin addicts, homosexuals, Haitians, and hemophiliacs). The earliest social representations largely portrayed the disease as a moral and social crisis above a health epidemic, positioning those infected as "deviant" in some way, thus framing the diagnosis as a consequence for homosexual behavior (LePoire, 1994; Páez et al., 1991; Sacks, 1996; Watney, 1989; Weeks, 1985). During this phase, media aired many conflicting reports on the cause of AIDS, even after it was discovered that the disease was caused by the HIV virus (Epstein, 1996). This stage of AIDS coverage featured confusion, denial, and uncertainty (Patton, 1990; Rogers, Dearing, & Chang, 1991).

The second phase, and central to this book, was the "moral panic" agenda. From 1982 to 1985, mass media progressively, yet rapidly, escalated conversations surrounding AIDS with tones of panic and fear (Weeks, 1989). This was the point at which public hysteria became apparent, with many media reports cultivating AIDS because of immoral (i.e., homosexual, non-masculine) sexual behavior (Joffe, 1995; Joffe, 1996). It is important to note that the hyperbolic scenarios used by media were not only present during this stage but seen throughout each era of AIDS coverage. AIDS stories were often driven as emergencies rather than long lasting concerns for public health, with attention-grabbing headlines privileged over attention to slow-onset issues (Dearing & Rogers, 1992; Sontag, 1988). Episodic framing was a common occurrence throughout the entire media coverage of AIDS, with news outlets rarely extending their storylines beyond panic and urgency to consider the larger socioeconomic contexts surrounding the disease (e.g., inequalities in treatment options, poverty as an influence on infection) (Emke, 2000). The encapsulation of short-term, life-or-death dramatic headlines became all too common in AIDS coverage as moral panic continued (Turoe & Coe, 1985).

The third phase (1985–1989) represented a period of "crisis management" (Weeks, 1989). Following the mass hysteria largely influenced by media, this period was marked by a more in-depth understanding of the effects of the crisis, whereby the disease was becoming more understood, yet misinformation surrounding marginalized populations was still apparent. Once media had planted the seed that heterosexual practices were the best protection from HIV/AIDS, it became difficult for science to play catch-up in changing the public's mind (Osborn, 1986). Following this phase, HIV/AIDS became routinized news stories with only periodic media triggering events (Swain, 2005). Now decades removed from mass hysteria, it is important to note that although science has made incredible strides in the treatment of AIDS, where individuals are now able to more proactively manage the disease, media coverage still creates frames. Coverage of AIDS beginning in the 1990s led the public to believe that it is all but cured (Cohen, 1997). That perception might exist in Western cultures that create "widespread complacency" (Swain, 2005, p. 259), but really, underdeveloped nations still battle the disease in great numbers, with nearly 37 million documented cases of HIV in 2017, including 1.8 million new diagnoses, that places the disease in a "prevention crisis" (Sidibé, 2018, p. 2). Media framing of the epidemic has evolved over time, however, from emphasizing a death sentence with the diagnosis to now presenting it as a chronic disease that can be better managed over time (Bardhan, 2001). While this frame is better aligned with scientific progression, the frequency of coverage still poses a problem. By 1994, 70 percent of media stories mentioning AIDS were reporting on something else altogether. As time has progressed, AIDS stories have become shorter and more focused on celebrities (Brodie et al., 2004). Perhaps most important to consider in this instance is not necessarily the drop in stories, which is somewhat expected as other health concerns are introduced on a global scale, but the degree to which AIDS coverage suffered a form of "compassion fatigue." In this sense, there has been a desensitization apparent in response to the social and emotional problems associated with AIDS that received so much attention throughout the 1980s and into the early 1990s (Kinnick, Krugman, & Cameron, 1996).

A discussion of media coverage of AIDS would be incomplete without acknowledging the role professional sports figures played in media framing of the disease. Jhally (1989) and McChesney (1989) have discussed the ways in which sport and mass media have participated in a mutually beneficial relationship, where mediated sports can act as cultural hegemony. Two examples of professional athletes who influenced the media's coverage of AIDS are Magic Johnson and Greg Louganis (Wachs & Dworkin, 1997). These examples offer the contradictory nature of media framing, especially when considering hegemonic masculinity in sport.

Johnson was a pillar for the NBA when he announced he was HIV-positive on November 7, 1991. A face of the "Showtime" Los Angeles

Lakers championship teams of the 1980s, Johnson fit the already masculine construction of sport in the United States. In analyzing coverage of his experience with HIV, media framed him as a hero for having lived with a stigmatized illness, one which he overemphasized was inflicted upon him through a heterosexual relationship (Cole & Denny, 1994; Payne & Mercuri, 1993; Wachs & Dworkin, 1997). In his initial announcement, he even explicitly stated that, if anything, he is "too heterosexual." The *Los Angeles Times* reported of the smiling, friendly Johnson, "You don't have to avoid Magic Johnson. He is not contaminated. He is not a leper. He is still Magic Johnson" (Downey, 1991, C1). Johnson's diagnosis was primarily positioned within the context of promiscuity in professional athletics to further situate him within hegemonic masculine discourse of sports reporting (Cole & Denny, 1994; Dworkin & Wachs, 1998).

Louganis, an Olympic diver who won gold medals for the United States in 1984 and 1988, revealed in a February 24, 1995, interview on the television news program *20/20* that he was HIV-positive and had been while competing in the 1988 Seoul Olympics (Nair, 2000). While media reports indicated "shock" at Johnson's announcement, conversely, that was not the case for Louganis, who had announced one year earlier that he was gay. Dworkin and Wachs (1998) explained that for media, Louganis's "homosexuality is a catch-all which signifies participation in high-risk activities, promiscuity, and inevitable contraction" (p. 8). Thus, he was framed as a carrier of the disease who was responsible for getting the disease. Within the discourse of hegemonic masculinity, sexuality was connected to each athlete's respective diagnosis, where Louganis was positioned as a "cause-and-effect" of homosexuality versus Johnson's accidental transmission through an unprotected, heterosexual encounter. Thus, awareness for his heterosexual partners and recognition that AIDS was not just a "gay" disease played prominently in media reports.

The only common feature in the framing of Johnson and Louganis was for possible risk of transmission through sport. Rather than place emphasis on Louganis's career accomplishments, as media did with Johnson, the focus became one incident of his bleeding in public after he hit his head on the diving board at the 1988 Olympics, which created mass hysteria whereby others could have been infected through transmission in the pool or to the team physician who treated him (Dorman, 2000; Nair, 2000; Wachs & Dworkin, 1997). When Johnson announced his retirement in 1991, other NBA players raised concern over whether they could have contracted the virus through contact on the basketball court. Johnson returned to compete as a member of the 1992 U.S. "Dream Team" at the Barcelona Olympics and for thirty-two games with the Lakers in 1996, but he retired again amid "homosocial" fear that ultimately expelled him from the masculine sport (Nair, 2000). Despite "negligible" risk of transmission during a sporting event, contact sports began to implement rules regarding visible blood and a need to disinfect both the athlete and his uniform before he could return to competition (Dorman, 2000). The juxtaposition of how Johnson and Louganis were framed by media offers an example of how media is positioned in the hegemonic masculine space created through sport and subsequent health concerns. Beyond diagnosis and cause, it becomes important to consider social and cultural implications when examining media coverage.

BIG TOBACCO AND SCIENTIFIC DOUBT

While HIV/AIDS offers a scientific example of an epidemic-led mediated public health concern (for which this book positions CTE at a similar level), Big Tobacco provides a long-term sociocultural shift in public perception and media framing that helps understand the NFL within the context of this book (Paolini, 2019). Although tobacco use was alive following the Civil War, subsequent advances in mass-production coupled with aggressive marketing presented an opportunity for the cigarette industry to be born. The cultural significance of cigarettes was apparent by the 1940s and into the early 1950s, with the addictive habit of smoking representing glamour, independence, and sociability (Rodrigues, 2009; Walsh-Childers, 2017). Countless celebrities, including Audrey Hepburn and Humphrey Bogart, smoked on- and off-screen, reaffirming the social acceptance of smoking in the public eye. Advertising campaigns such as Philip Morris's Marlboro Man or the Joe Camel cartoon helped to promote the idea that smoking cigarettes was cool, cheap, and socially acceptable (Rodrigues, 2009). Media framing of using tobacco and smoking has a long history in the United States, dating back as early as World War I. Cigarette smoking saw a significant boost once tobacco was rationed, with citizens even urged by major newspapers to support the war effort by supplying cigarettes for the soldiers overseas (Tate, 2000).

A monumental crisis for the tobacco industry began in 1950 when scientists Sir Richard Doll and A. Bradford Hill established in their research that smoking cigarettes caused lung cancer (Boseley, 2006; Doll & Hill, 1950). However, the public had not taken strong notice, likely because smoking's popularity and mediated glorification had just taken hold and the long-term effects were unknown. However, subsequent studies by Doll and Hill further validated their original findings (Doll & Hill, 1952, 1954, 1956) and created initial demand for public attention and government intervention. By the end of 1953, it became clear that scientific knowledge had reached a point of certainty regarding the link between smoking and lung disease, as well as other respiratory and cardiac diseases all leading to death (Brandt, 2012).

The progress science made in determining the detrimental effects of smoking did not align with the messages the tobacco industry had pushed on the public. The nomenclature of "Big Tobacco" was born following the industry's response to the public health crisis and speaks to its cultural and financial force as a conglomerate of strong corporations (Andelman, 1994). Rather than work with science, tobacco industry CEOs came together in an unprecedented move. They hired John W. Hill of the leading public relations firm Hill & Knowlton to design ways for the industry to combat the negative public image. Hill instructed the CEOs to take back control of science regarding tobacco. The goal became to design and disseminate a messaging strategy in direct response to the already-existing scientific findings. If Big Tobacco could effectively cast doubt upon the reliability and validity of the findings linking tobacco to lung cancer, they would simultaneously create a major scientific controversy by inserting their own version of science into the conversation (Brandt, 2012). Therefore, Big Tobacco launched its own scientific endeavor aimed at positioning the industry's assertion over what was perceived as an independent, scientifically verified knowledge domain. If successful, Big Tobacco could create a new arena ripe with conflicts of interest, "not for purposes of research and development but, rather, to undo what was now known: that cigarette smoking caused lethal disease" (Brandt, 2012, p. 64). Thus, the billion-dollar industry sought to "'unmake' a scientific fact" (Brandt, 2012, p. 64) through communication strategies aimed to discredit science and reaffirm public trust (Fleck, 1979; Proctor & Schiebinger, 2008; Wipfli & Samet, 2016).

Hill's strategy for Big Tobacco was to fabricate science rather than avoid it (Brandt, 2012). By instructing the CEOs to become avid supporters of science, it created a narrative whereby they also acknowledged the positive value of scientific skepticism, meaning that they perpetuated the notion that the effects of smoking remained an open question, as this fueled the controversy they sought to create (Brandt, 2007; Brandt, 2012; Michaels, 2008; Oreskes & Conway, 2010). Hill assembled a team of university-based scientists who were paid for supporting Big Tobacco's agenda. This team, referred to as the Tobacco Industry Research Committee (TIRC), convened in December 1953 and continued to participate in strategic and explicit collusion for more than five decades afterward (*United States v. Philip Morris* et al., 2004). The first step in TIRC's control of the narrative came soon after Hill was hired when the committee ran a full-page advertisement on January 4, 1954. The ad was placed in 448 U.S. newspapers under the heading "Frank Statement to Cigarette Smokers" that subsequently become known simply as the "frank statement" (Wipfli & Samet, 2016). The ad spoke directly to cigarette smokers and stated that the tobacco industry would begin aggressively pursuing "the science of tobacco" to ensure consumer well-being.

> We accept an interest in people's health as a basic responsibility, paramount to every other consideration in our business. We believe the products we make are not injurious to health. We always have and

> always will cooperate closely with those whose task it is to safeguard the public health. (Brandt, 2012; Tobacco Industry Research Committee, 1954)

Through its calculated public relations response, Big Tobacco was pushing another product to its consumers—doubt.

The TIRC secured academic support by forming the Scientific Advisory Board (SAB), comprised of academic researchers handpicked by Hill & Knowlton. The TIRC and SAB provided funding for research primarily focusing on cancer, while not directly addressing any of the medical risks associated with smoking (Brandt, 2012). Doing so aligned with the views of TIRC scientific director Clarence Cook Little, whom the tobacco industry had latched onto early in its public campaign. Little, a biologist and eugenicist who had strong views that cancer must be genetic and therefore not caused by smoking, helped to perpetuate the agenda of the tobacco industry in blurring the boundaries between public relations and science (Brandt, 2012; Pierce & Gilpin, 2001). Well into the 1960s, the TIRC had diverted enough attention away from the health risks associated with smoking to continue the manufactured controversy it had created. The TIRC and SAB presented perhaps the most well-known and documented instances of academic conflicts of interest with major corporations. What was most detrimental about this, however, was the ways in which these relationships and the information they created influenced media coverage of the issues (Pierce & Gilpin, 2001).

The TIRC constantly courted journalists, repeating its claims that the tobacco industry's priority was to public health. They continued to claim that the tobacco industry was skeptical of the science available at the time, which was reported by the media, thus potentially creating the same skepticism for individual media consumers (Brandt, 2007). Additionally, tobacco companies funneled millions in advertising dollars, and at times, received quid pro quo positive media coverage (McCandless, Yerger, & Malone, 2012). At the time that journalists were reporting on this, it is important to mention that they had little education or training on the scientific controversy, but by creating space for doubt, the public relations firm handed the media a pre-packaged story that had two clear opposing positions, further adding to the frame that tobacco science was "unresolved" (Brandt, 2012; Klaidman, 1991).

The public relations work of Hill and Knowlton was proven effective in looking at the rates of smoking—from 1954 to 1961, per capita consumption increased by almost one billion (Hill, Darrow, Thompson, & Hoyt, 1962). However, by the mid-1960s, enough scientists (including many on the SAB) had expressed enough skepticism that Big Tobacco could no longer hide behind the faulty science it had created. In 1964, the surgeon general released a damning report officially recognizing the harmful health risks associated with tobacco, at a time when 42 percent of

Americans still smoked (Keck, 2009). Tobacco consumption was undoubtedly linked to cancers, cardiovascular and respiratory diseases, adverse reproductive effects, and several other long-term health risks (Dutta & Boyd, 2007). The surgeon general's report paved a path for litigation and presented an opportunity for government intervention, thus causing an increase in the amount of tobacco lobbying seen in Washington (Keck, 2009). By 1965, Congress required that all cigarette packages have warning labels, and public education programs began to warn about the risks associated with smoking (Keck, 2009; Wipfli & Samet, 2016).

Broadcast media banned all cigarette advertising in 1971, which created a significant increase in cigarette advertising in print media (Dutta & Boyd, 2007). This is not to say that cigarettes did not have a place within broadcast media. Tobacco use was still featured for audiences through product placement and characters who smoked. Signorielli (1998) found that when characters on television smoked, they almost always exhibited positive traits, thus serving as role models (Signorielli, 1998). Smokers in popular films were also found to be more romantically and sexually active than nonsmokers (McIntosh, Bazzini, Smith, & Wayne, 1998). These findings were consistent with the fact that media coverage of health behaviors was more likely to positively portray unhealthy behaviors as opposed to emphasizing the associated negative consequences or risks (Heeter, Perlstadt, & Greenberg, 1984; Signorielli, 1990). However, positive mediated portrayals of smoking started to diminish. Wayne McLaren, the famous "Marlboro Man," developed lung cancer in the 1980s and began working as a spokesman for an anti-smoking campaign until he died in 1992 of cancer caused by smoking. By the mid-1990s, it appeared that the glamour and chicness once associated with cigarettes had finally worn off.

Big Tobacco started settling with individual states in 1997. Mississippi settled first, followed by Florida, Texas, and Minnesota. The four major U.S. tobacco companies were forced to publicly accept responsibility in 1998 with the Master Settlement Agreement, which ordered them to pay $206 billion across forty-six states, the largest settlement in United States history (Keck, 2009; Wander & Malone, 2006; Wipfli & Samet, 2016). The TIRC was forced to disband after the settlement. In 2008, after years of investigation, the U.S. Court of Appeals upheld a ruling which found the tobacco industry "guilty of engaging in a decades-long conspiracy to defraud the American public about the health risks of tobacco" (Keck, 2009, para. 16). In 2014, the major tobacco companies reached an agreement with the federal government to publish corrective statements addressing that Big Tobacco had lied about the harmful effects of smoking (Felberbaum, 2014; Walsh-Childers, 2017).

The Master Settlement Agreement banned cigarette product placement and most outdoor forms of advertising, yet the ads persisted in many print magazines (Dutta & Boyd, 2007; "Tobacco Master Settlement," 2001). An analysis of men's magazines from 2001 found that four predominant forms of masculinity were still apparent in portrayals of smoking in magazines: the sensual man, a man in an "other" place, the independent man, and the mysterious man (Dutta & Boyd, 2007). This shows the ways in which media continued to portray the positive, social aspects of smoking rather than acknowledging its unhealthy consequences and risk factors, which exemplifies the powerful force of masculinity. Ultimately, the case of Big Tobacco provides insight into the ways in which the industry and the media can influence public perception of health issues, but it also raises important opportunities for comparison in looking at media coverage of similar topics.

FRAMING AN EPIDEMIC

This chapter examined two case studies aimed at providing deeper context for the ways in which media succeeded and failed in recognizing public health hazards, particularly when having to consider multiple stakeholders (e.g., the public, corporate entities, celebrities). There is much to be learned from media framing of these instances and their respective influence on scientific understanding. HIV/AIDS is an infectious disease described as the "most devastating that humankind has ever faced" (Swain, 2005, p. 258). Tobacco "reflects perhaps the earliest example of the globalization of a noninfectious cause of disease" (Wipfli & Samet, 2016, p. 150). Thus, the contradiction and parallel of these global epidemics are important to understand when considering the issue of brain injuries and CTE in the NFL.

Overall, this case study approach emphasized the ways in which media and science are not intersecting, but rather, *parallel* forces that work alongside one another during times of public education. However, it is when these industries intersect, often centered around a crisis, where media begin to misinterpret scientific information packaged into narrative formats that increase readership and ratings. In the case of HIV/AIDS coverage, initial reports fueled public panic and misinformation. It was only once media "calmed down" and began really digesting the existing science behind HIV/AIDS that the public could then be properly educated for the first time on the issue. Here, the science was crucial in calming the public's fears with media as the vehicle responsible for getting this information out.

This chapter outlined how media framing works and emphasizes the influence media can have both in creating public awareness and panic, especially when intersecting with science, as well as influencing policy and perception. It is important to recognize that media provide a powerful and influential role in how it constructs messages, but those messages are presented by and through government, organizations, and individuals. Thus, this book recognizes the significance of media framing as a process of social construction in how an entire issue is understood (Carter, 2013). However, this research does not examine all the various availability entrepreneurs involved in the construction of knowledge nor how individuals interpret the mediated information about CTE and the NFL. As Iyengar and Kinder (1987) recognized "surely viewers are influenced not only by the amount of news but also by the *kind* of news" (p. 35). Therefore, this book explores what kind of news is selected in the reporting of CTE to examine media for its complex role as both participant in the process and producer of frames that serve as a site of struggle over how CTE, and by extension the NFL, is framed (Gamson & Modigliani, 1989; Gurevitch & Levy, 1985) and the responses from the NFL and other significant social institutions. Over the next two chapters, a brief history of the NFL and its foundation in masculinity is outlined to better understand how and why CTE gained a meteoric rise in public attention to set up the media framing study that was conducted in this book.

THREE

Hegemonic Masculinity

The Foundation of American Football Culture

American football has permeated beyond its base of diehard sports fans and pushed itself into social realms once reserved for conversations and activities unrelated to sports such as politics and religion. As Newkirk (2017) explained, "football is the way Americanness is performed now" (para. 7). Football is interwoven into a media landscape embedded in a fan culture that has used mediated experience as a coping mechanism for daily life (Lewis, 1992; Oates, 2017). The mediated significance of the NFL—and other professional sports leagues—shifted in the 1980s when most team owners generated more revenue from television contracts than ticket sales, and this economic growth paralleled a push in American capitalism (Teitelbaum, 2010). Sport consumption for fans was no longer relegated to experience only in the sporting arena. Instead, people could share the mediated experience through television and rehash the game in the office. This cultural significance has moved to debating the success or failure of a football team, either real or fantasy, in virtual and online spaces (Bell, Morales, & Robb, 2017). No matter where someone turned, football often entered the conversation.

The growth of football in the United States has transformed how people engage and interact with each other, especially on Sunday afternoons. Once a day devoted to church and other religious activities, observance has been challenged—and at times replaced—by pigskin and hard hits. Football has been defined as a ritualized process that is performed by players, guided by coaches, perpetuated by media, and unconsciously attended and adored by fans that collaborate as a socializing agent under the control of masculinity (Axelrod, 2001; Sabo & Panepinto, 1990). It is as though the experience and its associated rituals where masculinity, especially violence displayed in and through sport, becomes a culturally accepted norm, almost part of a daily routine. Yet, despite its Sunday takeover, the growth in football's popularity was a gradual, historical process that culturally developed over time, with media as a beneficial conduit between player and fan (Oriard, 1993).

Football has and continues to evolve into a sport with the power to dictate trends, especially in popular culture (Danesi, 2012; Kennedy & Hills, 2009). Media interest to showcase the sport's top players on a weekly basis contributes to a growing obsession with football that raises athletes to exalted levels in society (Keith, 2010). However, the game that grew through its visual depiction of mediated violence faces a shift in cultural values that continue to be challenged, especially as new information is revealed related to head injuries (Oriard, 2014a). Thus, better understanding of the long-term risk and repercussions from participation in contact sport is called for in response to the masculine ideal to play through pain at all costs (Sabo, 2009). The NFL has responded with rule changes made at the league's discretion that serve to push an agenda that positions the league with a goal of putting player safety first, which through historical analysis of lawsuits and stories in the popular press was not always a league mantra. This perceived ideological shift is discussed later, but first, it is significant to define hegemonic masculinity and how it ascribes to football.

HEGEMONIC MASCULINITY AND VIOLENCE

Thought of separately, hegemony is a socializing process aimed at winning control of power, often through ideological means and not necessarily force (Bates, 1975; Donaldson, 1993). Masculinity relates to a gendered order of sex roles positioned as normative male values. Sexton (1969) prescribed some of these values as "courage, inner direction, certain forms of aggression, autonomy, mastery, technological skill, group solidarity, adventure, and a considerable amount of toughness in mind and body" (p. 15). Donaldson (1993) explains that "heterosexuality and homophobia are the bedrock of hegemonic masculinity" (p. 645) to situate gendered norms of male as dominant and powerful in an oppressive relationship to women and other groups perceived as subordinate. Thus, hegemonic masculinity can be understood as a process to recirculate and adapt to new modes of maintaining power within a defined social structure that initially created power in favor of men (Carrigan, Connell, & Lee, 1985).

If heterosexuality and homophobia provide a bedrock of hegemonic masculinity, then violence and pain offer a bedrock of American football that firmly situates its place as a purveyor of hegemonic masculinity (Sabo, 2009; Stade, 1966). Thus, hegemonic masculinity and American football are ideologically intertwined (Sanderson, Weathers, Grevious, Tehan, & Warren, 2016) as a space created by and perpetuated for men, as it is the only sanctioned sport without a significant female counterpart. When considering Sexton's values of masculinity within football, mediated notions of courage are positioned alongside aggression, mastery, solidarity, and toughness to idealize what a football player should be. Whether connected to toughness, strength, or violence, football and other contact sports are associated with harm (McNamee, 2014) where a need to play through pain is expected (Anderson & Kian, 2012), normalized by the media (McGannon, Cunningham, & Schinke, 2013), and a form of exploitation promulgated by sport (Murphy & Waddington, 2007).

American football has evolved from a sport that closely mirrored rugby into one with its own set of rules and regulations aimed to distinguish itself from its sporting predecessor. Over time, many changes have occurred to both the rules of the sport and equipment used by the players that have been influenced through governmental intrusion aimed, at least on the surface, to improve player safety. Instead, "changes were not fundamental" (Heinze & Lu, 2017, p. 505), but were simply organizational responses to institutional pressures. Football leadership has never willingly altered the violent nature of the sport. It has only done so when external forces applied enough pressure, and even then, it is questionable as to what the hopeful outcome would provide.

President Roosevelt's involvement in 1905 to reform the sport, for example, has been hypothesized as something more than aimed at helping save lives that were being lost through the sport that did not reward players with the financial riches of the twenty-first century (Gordon, 2014). As Guttmann (2006) outlined, "Roosevelt, a great believer in football as a school of masculinity, intervened, not to abolish football but to save it from abolition" (p. 538). While the extreme (e.g., death) was the mediated focus for Roosevelt, what was not discussed was how the violent nature of football that he claimed to remedy was—and always has been—embedded in the notion of hegemonic masculinity. In its basic form, football men were autonomous to change the social structure of the sport for the betterment of men, despite its violent underpinnings.

More than fifty years ago, Stade (1966) opined that football "is one whose mode is violence and whose violence is its special glory" (p. 40). Thus, anything less than machismo and bravado is considered weak, especially regarding injuries, and does not fit into the masculine ideal to "shake it off," "rub some dirt on it," or "get back in there" despite the possible long-term effects, especially with repeated blows to the head in high-impact sport. Return-to-play guidelines hope to remove autonomy from a player or coach into the direction of the medical decision-makers to determine a player's readiness to return to the game (Bowers, 2014; Darrow, Collins, Yard, & Comstock, 2009; Fedderman-Dermont, Straumann, & Dvořák, 2014; McClincy, Lovell, Pardini, Collins, & Spore, 2006), but the socialized mentality of hegemonic masculinity embedded in football creates a difficult space to enforce these criteria that were constructed outside the control of football decision-makers.

In his study about masculinity in Canadian football, which is American football played on a larger field, Fogel (2011) addressed how players can exert their power because of their place and identity within sport and society. Because "football remains as one of the last male spaces in the sports coliseum" (Fogel, 2011, p. 12), men are often given a pass regarding violent acts. Viewing football as a "dying breed" suggests the last thing men want to do is surrender their power or share their space with women, especially given the societal constructs of gender roles. Therefore, to maintain their position, violent behavior is expected and unfortunately accepted as part of a normalized football culture both on and off the field (Adubato, 2016; Axelrod, 2001; Beissel, Giardina, & Newman, 2014; Guttmann, 2006; Messner, 1990; Welch, 1997). These studies identified mass media as an effect through the glorification of the sporting violence that transfers beyond the game.

Fogel (2011) goes a step further to create a subcategory of hegemonic masculinity, which he calls sporting masculinity. He suggests that hegemonic masculinity serves as an umbrella term that defines a pecking order among men, while sporting masculinity allows room for men to be marginalized within the sport. This marginalization can be a by-product of how a head coach exerts controls where players are systematically instructed to conform to masculine ideals through deference and pain that simultaneously extols the virtues of manhood and denigrates notions of femininity (Guttmann, 2006; Sabo & Panepinto, 1990). Often masculinity negatively influence players' off-field behavior. These acts of violent exertion—having to constantly be tough and superior—have led to numerous off-the-field issues, primarily acts of violence against women, including rape and other forms of sexual assault and harassment. Media have played a role in defending these violent acts through the narrative ways they frame victims (Waterhouse-Watson, 2013). Thus, the violence created in a "sports so dependent upon raw force" (Stade, 1966, p. 40) cannot be ignored as it extends to all forms of football culture (e.g., American, Australian, Canadian).

USA Today maintains a database of NFL player arrests dating to 2000. Through the end of June 2018, the database counted 897 incidents where players were arrested, charged, and/or convicted of crimes, which averages to approximately fifty per year. Driving under the influence charges account for more than one-fourth of the arrests (n = 241, 26.9 percent). When considering that, sadly, nearly one million people are arrested every year in the United States for DUI, the NFL number does not appear too large. However, of the remaining 656 arrests, more than one-third (n = 249, 38 percent) were for some type of violent act. Domestic violence (n = 107) and assault (n = 83) accounted for most of these arrests. The remaining charges were for battery (*n* = 23), sexual assault or other sex charges (*n* = 16), animal abuse or cruelty (*n* = 8), murder or manslaughter (*n* = 8), child abuse (*n* = 3), and pimping (*n* = 1).

As the numbers indicate, some examples moved beyond violent attacks to deadly encounters embedded in the sporting masculinity culture. Multiple players have been charged with (e.g., Ray Lewis, O. J. Simpson) or convicted of murder (e.g., Rae Carruth, Aaron Hernandez, Eric Naposki, Robert Rozier) or committed murder before suicide (e.g., Jovan Belcher). These acts of deadly rage are further complicated when considering the trauma inflicted on these players' bodies and brains invariably caused by their sport. Clearly this is no justification for the violent way they took another human being's life. However, it does speak to a willingness to hide the impact of violence as accepted practice in these sports.

The repetitive collisions endured specifically by football players have been studied to determine the impact on an athlete's psyche. Welch (1997) explored how the violence players exhibit during the game is sometimes carried over into their personal lives. Since football is played in a space that enables "controlled violence" (p. 393), the perception is that a player should be able to differentiate that behavior and isolate it to the sporting space. However, Welch and other scholars found that this violence extends past the field and is inclusive of non-football-related activities that sports leagues claim to address through collective bargaining and suspensions but has increased public concern largely through media representations (Brown, Murphy, & Maxwell, 2018; Enck-Wanzer, 2009; McDonald, 1999; Pappas, McKenry, & Catlett, 2004; Posthuma, Flores, Barlow, & Dworkin, 2018).

Turning off this violent mentality may be difficult as they have been trained and socialized to take orders and perform malicious acts as part of their daily work routine (Kimmel & Messner, 1992). As Schneider and Eitzen (2010) hypothesized, "perhaps football allows too much 'legitimate' body contact for an athlete's own safety" (p. 417). The effect of violence in the sport "workplace" is comparable to that of war veterans who must transition from violence abroad on a battlefield to civilian life at home. The narrative crossover of violence and hegemonic masculinity in sport and war has a longstanding tradition that is perpetuated by mediated metaphors that overlap the language of war journalists and sports media (Jansen & Sabo, 1994; Kellett, 2002). Thus, examining football's relationship to war is critical to understand, as it may offer some foundation for the masculine ideology embedded in football culture.

FOOTBALL AND/AS WAR

The correlation between football and war transcended geographic boundaries but has often been connected to the World Wars, especially for the

Allied Powers of Britain and the United States. Both institutions were known for an ability to mobilize large groups of young men to fight for a nation or team. As Burstyn (1999) explained for the British Empire there was a parallel rise of British militarization around the first World War and men's sports, where "military and athletic institutions overlapped and interpenetrated, and their cultures evolved in tandem" (p. 67). Burstyn described a similar rise in the United States in the late nineteenth century alongside the commercialization of professional sports and increased military expenditures where this process provided "a way to succeed in the noble enterprise of nation-building and nation-extending war" (p. 67).

Montez de Oca (2013) produced an insightful account of the rise to prominence of college football during the Cold War as a reification of masculine identity to battle against both the Soviets and the feminization of American culture. He paid special attention to the role of media in co-constructing this narrative. Oates (2017) outlined how the NFL, following the merger with the AFL, built its empire as a "commercial force" (p. 11) by capitalizing on similar ideas of American exceptionalism produced by college football during wartime. The creation of new forms of mass media worked to amplify and circulate a "glorification of warfare" (Messner, 2012, p. 119) linked with masculinity and nationalism in sport. Butterworth (2017) reinforced the institutional parallels of military and sport in the twenty-first century as marketed ideals often re-inscribed by and through media.

It was not just media that worked to build this bridge between football and war. On January 11, 1961, Robert Kennedy, just nine days before he started his role as U.S. attorney general, said to a gathering of college coaches in New York, "Except for war, there is nothing in American life—nothing—which trains a boy better for life than football" (Clinch, 1973, p. 266). This quote offered a unique perspective from the former Harvard football player and member of the U.S. Navy during a time of social turbulence in the United States, Clinch (1973) noted that Kennedy later changed his opinion about war but added that the football/war comparison creates a "belief in the masculine mystique of physical toughness" (p. 266). Kennedy's quote has been widely recirculated as an exemplary parallel for football and war in connection with masculine ideology (Ball, 2000; Burgess, Edwards, & Skinner, 2003; Fields, 2008; Kemper, 2009).

A look at magazine and newspaper headlines can reinforce the commonalities that football and war share centered around violence.

> "Ready for some football, and war?"
>
> —*The Washington Post*, January 12, 2003
>
> "War is hell—but this is football."
>
> —*San Mateo County Times*, January 21, 2003

"Football lessons recalled in war."

—*USA Today*, August 18, 2004

"Football as war and an American obsession."

—*Denver Examiner*, January 26, 2013

"Football is America's war game."

—*The Los Angeles Times*, August 23, 2014

"Football has always been a battleground in the culture war."

—*The Atlantic*, September 29, 2017

These headlines speak to a parallel that can define football as uniquely American. Stade (1966) provided a comparison to the ideological underpinning of the nation's founding fathers through aggressive defense of territory. He asked, "Does this not make football *par excellence* the game of instinctual satisfaction among Americans, who are notorious as violent patriots and instinctive defenders of private property?" (p. 41). The ultimate outcome for both football and war is winning, where sacrifice is a foundational pillar perpetuated by media (Sage, 1998). The hard-hitting collisions and competitive spirit determine who is the last man standing, which helps support the idea that to earn victory the opponent must suffer. The war-like violent nature of football and its widespread acceptance is thus normalized as a likely outcome despite evidence of long-term effects often overlooked by leagues and media members who fuel the ideology of sporting masculinity (Washington & Karen, 2010).

For example, in making the case that football equals war, Edmundson (2014) uses language that paints a picture for anyone unfamiliar with football, yet clearly aware of a militaristic vision of violence and combat.

> Football is a tank attack, a sky-borne assault, a charge into the trenches for hand-to-hand fighting. Football is following orders and sticking to the strategy; it's about acting as a unit and taking hits for the group. Football is generals (coaches) and captains (quarterbacks) and the enlisted guys who play on the line. Football is about destruction . . . you generally have to slam the life out of your opponents. You try to do away with their skill players—by violence. (para. 10 & 11)

A reader can envision a general/coach giving orders/plays to his captain/quarterback for their march/drive down the field. These orders/plays are then relayed to the rest of the unit/team, whose task is to work in unison to defeat the enemy/opponent and ultimately, secure a victory.

Edmundson's work is just one example of how language can be used to invoke an image of war which like sports served as a growth stimulus for news media (Bell, 1991; Boyce, Curran, & Wingate, 1978). Groothuis (2014) wrote about football and its undeniable violence, likening the players' pads to that of armor with a likely outcome of multiple injuries in battle, noting that, "Yes, players of any contact sport risk injury, but not in the same sense as the millionaire gladiators of the gridiron. In no other sport must the contestants wear body armor. But even that armor cannot cover the carnage" (para. 7). Again, the language is meant to compare the roles of football players to that of soldiers at war. They are donning equipment meant to protect them in battle, yet that same equipment can only protect against minor combat pain because they are always at risk of permanent damage. This win-at-all-cost mentality feeds into what Sabo (2009) defined as the "pain principle," which is "a patriarchal cultural belief that pain is inevitable and that the endurance of pain enhances one's character and moral worth" (p. 146), and it is rooted in masculine social organizations like military and sport.

Injuries often overlooked due to desire for acceptance in the hegemonic masculine space have long-term effects, sometimes without revealing significant impact for years or even decades after an initial injury. It is during this time when athletes are often left to navigate these post-career injuries alone despite a desire to play through pain to avoid being stigmatized within masculine ideals (Washington & Karen, 2010; Young et al., 1994). This is yet another similarity to soldiers who experience flashbacks and other post-traumatic events following their return from deployment and, at times, receive limited medical care for mental health issues (Hester, 2017). Essentially, the violence men inflict upon each other throughout their career may help explain why some are unable to avoid replicating this behavior off the field.

In recent years, recognition of debilitating mental effects has begun to get recognized by these social institutions beyond the pain principle associated with bodily harm. The military has produced a similar lineage to football with CTE in its varying terminology to define long-term neurological effects of combat. The descriptions range from "shell shock" to "battle fatigue" to "posttraumatic stress disorder" (PTSD). Each one describes the physical and psychological toll suffered from injuries sustained in combat (Reid & Velez, 2015). Additionally, it is significant to note that long-term effects are rarely caused by one instance of brain trauma. They are compiled through participation in a hazardous work environment where symptoms can vary to complicate accurate medical diagnoses (Lew, Otis, Tun, Kerns, Clark, & Cifu, 2009). Known as the "polytrauma clinical triad" in military linguistics, this trio of symptoms are chronic pain, TBI, and PTSD, and they rarely appear in isolation from the other symptoms. This cluster of symptoms is linked to violent impulses as well (Blakey et al., 2018). Thus, the parallel between football and war has transferred from foundational ideological constructs to scientific and linguistic overlap with media as a key player in engaging public discourse (Reid & Velez, 2015). However, simple recognition of long-term effects is not enough to challenge a stranglehold that hegemonic masculinity has on American social institutions. Instead, it is the duty of those who implement and uphold institutional policy and practice that must forge ahead to produce a cultural shift, which in the case of the NFL, has been met with resistance, especially toward commissioner Roger Goodell, who has been at the epicenter of most of the league's mediated controversies, including domestic violence and rule changes aimed at the sport's masculine domain.

CULTURE SHIFT

On August 8, 2006, Goodell was appointed NFL commissioner. Since his tenure began, more than fifty rule changes have been implemented, many of which were introduced under the guise to increase player safety (Myers, 2016; Seifert, 2016b). Seifert (2016b) notes that real changes were noticeable three years into Goodell's role as commissioner after "Goodell was grilled at a 2009 congressional hearing about the league's refusal to acknowledge a connection between brain injuries and football" (para. 6). Following this, Goodell shifted his focus, as well as that of the league, to preventing unnecessary head injury by developing, implementing, or tweaking rules to protect defenseless players. While this was a step in the right direction, some fans and players were not accepting of these changes.

In 2013, after proposing "offensive players cannot lead with the crown-of-the-helmet into defenders when outside of the tackle box" (Starkey, 2013, para. 1), fans took to Twitter to express their frustration with Goodell and new NFL rules focused on player safety. In 2016, when Goodell considered ejecting players from a game for receiving a *second* personal foul, Seattle Seahawks cornerback Richard Sherman voiced his displeasure during an interview on ESPN's *Sportscenter* on March 20, 2016:

> I think it's foolish. . . . But it sounds like something somebody who's never played the game would say, something that they would suggest, because he doesn't understand. He's just a face. He's just a suit. He's never stepped foot on the field and understood how you can get a personal foul. (Kapadia, 2016, para. 3)

Sherman's quote is situated within the notion of sporting masculinity to demean the commissioner for his lack of participation in and understanding of what it takes to play the sport. The quote was widely recirculated internationally by other media outlets (Condotta, 2016; Graham, 2016; Samuel, 2016). Despite the objections from players and fans alike regarding new and/or updated policies, rule changes have been—and continue to be—implemented to ensure the long-term health of players, and by extension, the NFL's valuable labor pool.

Sherman's thoughts on Goodell reflect a player culture that has gone as far as to state a willingness to die playing football and a fan culture that appreciates the violence witnessed every week (Crepeau, 2017). For example, at a press conference in the summer of 2017 at a New York Jets fan forum, rookie safety Jamal Adams, sitting next to Goodell, was asked about rule changes in the NFL and player safety. Adams best summed up that a shift in how some players view American football culture is anything but "soft" and a little disturbing.

> I can speak for a lot of the guys that play the game. We live and breathe (football) and this is what we're so passionate about. Literally, I would, if I had a perfect place to die, I would die on the field. I would be at peace. ("Jamal Adams," 2017)

Sadly, the 150 fans in attendance applauded Adams's statement, which speaks to the embedded culture of American football from the field to the stands. While Adams acknowledged his concern for player safety, his approach to playing football maintains a masculine identity handed down through generations of players such as Hall of Fame running back Earl Campbell, who mocked current NFL players for lacking the ability to play a game because of "a hangnail on my toe. . . . I didn't get a pedicure this week. I don't play because my head hurt" (Peter, 2017, para. 8). Campbell, who played eight seasons for the Houston Oilers and New Orleans Saints between 1978 and 1985, added that these excuses "wouldn't have got the job done back in my day" (Peter, 2017, para. 9) and thus, would not have been appreciated nor respected during his era.

Campbell's damning of the state of American football reaffirms the hold of masculine mentality on the sport and reinforces the pain principle as something to strive for and maintain for the sanctity of the sport. Anderson and Kian (2012) addressed this hegemonic masculine discourse that being soft in football is inappropriate and unacceptable, and that men are persuaded "to position their own bodies as an expendable weapon of athletic war" (p. 155). Thus, a player who chooses to do the opposite of what is expected of a manly player does not possess a masculine identity. Additionally, they are positioned outside the culture of toughness that requires, and even demands, a play-through-pain mentality (King et al., 2014; Nowinski, 2007; Young et al., 1994).

Even when not addressing injuries sustained on the field and the pain principle, mediated discourses reify the hegemonic masculine hold of football. These instances occur through a range of emotions from victimization in domestic violence cases (Oates, 2017) to celebrating participation over performance. For example, fans on Twitter responded to running back Adrian Peterson's suspension for child abuse and that the league's response was part of the "wussification" of America's sport that feeds on violence (Foote, Butterworth, & Sanderson, 2017). Another example of challenging manhood was when Pittsburgh Steelers linebacker James Harrison expressed his displeasure with his sons receiving "participation trophies" for their on-the-field efforts and not for winning. Harrison felt the trophies were undeserved and shared his frustration on Instagram:

> I came home to find out that my boys received two trophies for nothing, participation trophies! While I am very proud of my boys for everything they do and will encourage them till the day I die, these trophies will be given back until they EARN a real trophy. I'm sorry I'm not sorry for believing that everything in life should be earned (Boren, 2015, para. 4).

Harrison further explained these trophies are only meant to appease athletes who whine and complain to "shut u (sic) up and keep you happy" (Boren, 2015a, para. 4). Debate over trophies given to youth athletes teeters on supporting further participation versus rewarding achievement (Anshel, 2016). Harrison's comments suggest that manhood should not equate to effort in sport but to winning and dominance, and it fits his mediated persona. Beyond his social media rant, Harrison has been positioned at the unique intersection of mediated, violent celebrity through his nickname "The Hitman" but also as a voice of contestation against Goodell and the commissioner's unfair levying of fines from new rules, especially those fines against Black players. For a *Men's Journal* cover photo, Harrison was featured wielding two of his favorite guns that Beissel et al. (2014) described as a process that situated Harrison in a sports-war nexus as a narrative often extended by the sports media.

SPORTS MEDIA, INJURY, AND RESPONSIBILITY

American football is at an interesting crossroad centered on the media/sports complex that cannot find balance between valorizing the combat of football against the backdrop of player injuries. Oates (2017) asked, "What does the NFL stand for in contemporary U.S. media culture?" (p. 6). Conversely, we ask, what does media stand for in its long-standing relationship with the NFL? The master narrative gets muddied in a possible cultural shift in American football from masculinity to responsibility (Benson, 2017). The entertainment value of football—the team rivalries, hard hits, and halftime performances—offers a chance to engage socially in mediated "fun" for fans. However, the inherent violence in the sport makes it difficult for some to fully enjoy the viewing experience, knowing that a hit may injure a player, and perhaps kill him. American football culture has evolved from a game with little-to-no protection to a game whose focus—if one is to believe the NFL messaging—is shifting toward protecting its players. Yet, despite the publicized efforts by the NFL to make the game safer, there are suggestions that the league has simply co-opted the process by partnering with scientists and large corporations to create a public perception that is highly privatized as a form of organization power (Heinze & Lu, 2017).

Sports media have historically found itself trapped in the construction and re-inscription of hegemonic masculinity (Sabo & Panepinto, 1990). Journalists often follow an ideological construct that highlights strength, independence, and authority in describing positive attributes for men (van Dijk, 2009), and this is especially true in sports coverage. Media have helped normalize injury, pain, and risk in sport (Nixon, 1993). However, this historical lineage was mostly reserved for the athlete's body, not the brain. This is not to justify that it should be acceptable to minimize long-term destruction of the body. However, shifting the mediated discourse of risk to the mind has started to influence the previous glorification of football by and through media, especially when the injury involves a recognizable athlete, such as the quarterback position in the NFL (Anderson & Kian, 2012; McGannon et al., 2013).

Pittsburgh Steelers quarterback Ben Roethlisberger, for example, has been central in the mediated battle between affirming the sport's masculine ideology when considering head injuries. In a December 2, 2015, article in the *Washington Post*, ironically written by a female, the article points out that after a helmet-to-helmet hit that Roethlisberger, "whose history shows *a gutsy willingness* to play through pain" (Boren, 2015, emphasis added), remained on the field for a few plays but then "*took himself out* of the game" (Boren, 2015, emphasis added) for further examination. Later in the article, Roethlisberger is referred to as "one of the *toughest* players in the game" (Boren, 2015, emphasis added). The masculine ideals of gutsy and tough as well as the independent authority to remove one's self from the game situate Roethlisberger's autonomy as a male athlete.

The story did discuss how a star player's awareness of possible head trauma and willingness to exit the playing field is a positive step in recognition of possible long-term harm and newfound emphasis on player safety. However, the way the article portrays the athlete still adheres to the masculine principles associated with contact sport and is an example of how news values for journalists can be "contradictory and incoherent" (O'Neill & Harcup, 2009, p. 168). Roethlisberger's concussion also migrated into the role of health communication and accurate sharing of information between various medical professionals, which can be a key hurdle in accurate diagnosis, treatment, and hopeful recovery (Zasler, 2015). Thus, this story serves as an example for how journalists can share responsibility for player safety while, at the same time, re-inscribing the masculine ideology of American football.

Limited research has examined the role of media in constructing a narrative specific to brain injuries. Two studies centered on the role of media in discussing quarterbacks removing themselves from a game (Anderson & Kian, 2012; Sanderson et al., 2016). The quarterbacks in question were Jay Cutler, Robert Griffin III, and Aaron Rodgers. Overall, the findings indicate more signs of support from media for the player's autonomy. However, there was some blame placed on the athlete for an unwillingness to sacrifice his health for the success of the team. However, these findings cannot be applied to all NFL players because these studies were limited to the marquee position and players, who at the time of the studies, were entrenched as an unquestioned starter and possible franchise quarterback.

In a study of how concussions were framed in reporting on espn.com, Karimipour and Hull (2017) noted that concussions were "minimized, not medicalized" (p. 61) and discussed as everyday injuries that trivialized the potential harm different from other bodily injuries. This ambivalent type of reporting can lead to a mitigation of NFL responsibility (Sanderson et al., 2016). Ahmed and Hall (2017) identified descriptors for brain injuries in online news reporting across four sports (football, hockey, soccer, rugby) spanning five countries (United States, Canada, New Zealand, British Isles, Australia) as well as how concussions are positioned in relation to other neurodegenerative diseases. The authors noted a linguistic difference in how countries described these injuries, but "concussion" was used overwhelmingly, followed by either head or brain in conjunction with injury or trauma. CTE was discussed as the mention most frequently associated because of concussions.

However, it was beyond the findings that the authors provided the most insight for journalists reporting on sports injuries specific to the head. They offered a six-step "media concussion reporting checklist" to avoid tropes in reporting misinformation or improperly contextualizing the severity of injuries to the brain. These steps can be condensed to three primary ideological objectives. First, they noted that concussions are serious and that a more accurate medical description would be "brain injury" and to avoid sporting terms such as "ding" or "head clash." Second, modifiers (e.g., mild, severe) are misleading when used alongside concussion and should not be perpetuated by allowing players or coaches to describe the severity of a brain injury. Third, journalists must recognize that concussions should adhere to return-to-play guidelines and do not require a loss of consciousness. Adhering to this type of guideline could assist media in less valorization and glorification and more accurate detailed accounts of invisible injuries.

Academic research is not exempt from favoring these same masculine principles, especially when comparing a sport where participants cross gender boundaries. Despite female athletes showing a greater propensity for concussions than males in similar sports (Gessel, Fields, Collins, Dick, & Comstock, 2007), the difference in soccer is attributed to the "*smaller* size and *weaker* neck strength for female athletes to a *more aggressive male* athlete who is playing a faster-paced sport" (Schatz & Moser, 2011, p. 1044, emphasis added). While mainstream media and research have a way to go for equality, research delving into long-term cognitive impairment is valuable and a significant step toward cultural recognition. Concussions, CTE, and brain injuries in sports, with American football as the headline leader, have received significant media attention (Bowers, 2014; McGannon et al., 2013; Sanderson et al., 2016; Schatz & Moser, 2011; Zasler, 2015) that has sparked conversation on the front pages, in the courtrooms (Goldberg, 2013; Moser & Miller, 2014), and within the pages of academic and medical literature (Fedderman-Dermont et al., 2014; Gardner et al., 2014; McNamee, 2014; Omalu et al., 2005; Wojtys, 2016).

Though a masculine ideal to win-at-all-costs is a historical football framework, recent years have seen a shift in how potential long-term effects related to brain injuries are viewed by players who are exerting their greatest level of autonomy. During the 2015 NFL offseason, five players across three teams, all under thirty years of age, chose to retire. Three of these players played for the San Francisco 49ers—linebackers Chris Borland and Patrick Willis and offensive tackle Anthony Davis. Jake Locker played quarterback for the Tennessee Titans and Jason Worilds was a linebacker with the Steelers ("Early retirement," 2015). Early retirement is not uncommon in the NFL, evident by the average length of an NFL career shrunk from 4.99 years to 2.66 years between 2006 and 2014 (Arthur, 2016). However, Borland's retirement after earning all-rookie honors sent shockwaves through the sport and, subsequently, media. Just twenty-four at the time of his retirement, Borland was clear about what motivated his decision.

> I just want to do what's best for my health. . . . From what I've researched and what I've experienced, I don't think it's worth the risk. . . . I feel largely the same, as sharp as I've ever been, for me, it's about wanting to be proactive. . . . I'm concerned that if you wait till you have symptoms, it's too late (Middlehurst-Schwarz, 2015, para. 3 & 6)

Borland faced criticism *and* received praise as central to the debate whether he retired too young or took control of the situation before it got out of hand (Middlehurst-Schwartz, 2015). Borland was comfortable with his decision, as he knew it was the best for him to leave the "dehumanizing" profession (Benson, 2017; Oates, 2017), and he rejected the idea of coaching "because I wouldn't want to be charged with the task of making violence safer" (Fainaru & Fainaru-Wada, 2015, para. 15)

Players are becoming more concerned about their health, led by veterans who have dealt with head trauma and can serve as advocates for the player's union to challenge the hegemonic masculine ideology (Benton, 2017; Vrentas, 2017). Roethlisberger has spoken out on several occasions urging players to self-report their injuries. Despite his questionable off-the-field decisions that position him in the masculine ideology perpetuated through football (Beissel et al., 2014), Roethlisberger, who has sustained several injuries, including concussions, throughout his career, emphasized that the brain is one body part that can't be replaced, and should therefore, be treated with care (Benton, 2017). Similarly, Rodgers recounted two concussions from the 2010 season, especially one that he was later informed about:

> I got up . . . and my chinstrap was across my nose. You could see Gene Steratore, one of my favorite referees, and he kind of comes over to me, and he's like, "Hey, are you OK?" I don't remember this, but I'm like, "Yeah, I'm fine. I'm fine." There was a timeout called, went over to the sideline, and I think I waved off, "Oh, I'm good. I'm good." It's just kind of what's built into you. . . . I went back out there for a couple plays, and I couldn't call the plays, and they ended up getting me out of there. (Wood, 2016, para. 14 & 15)

Six years after the injury, Rodgers was able to laugh it off. However, Rodgers's attempt to continue playing reaffirms the narrative of playing through pain. His story, and lack of recollection, highlights a need for players to speak out or risk long-term health consequences.

Myles Garrett understood the risk and was willing to speak up, despite his perceived "rookie" status, which historically provides a space to show up and shut up. The number one overall pick by the Cleveland Browns in 2017, Garrett self-reported a concussion suffered against the Tennessee Titans on October 22 (Schad, 2017). The defensive end was criticized for reporting his injury, but when asked why he chose to report his injury, given the criticism he faced afterward, Garrett responded by pushing back against the notion of masculinity in American football, especially regarding brain injuries.

> It doesn't really bother me what other people say, whether I'm "being a man" or not. . . . I'll play through my foot, my arm, anything that's affecting me below my neck. I can't play around with my brain. . . . If it had been something like I guess something physical in my body, that's different. But you don't want to mess with your mind. . . . That's something that you can't get back. That's something you can't heal (Schad, 2017, para. 2 & 4)

Garrett's approach to self-reporting is critical and offers a counter-narrative to Adams's willingness to die on the field, as it signals that some players recognized, first and foremost, the importance of protecting their brain. Thus, Garrett exemplifies a slow shift toward self-reporting, which could indicate that medical research subsequently distributed by journalists emphasizes the importance of addressing head trauma in the face of hegemonic masculinity.

Yet, while a noble gesture, some athletes are hesitant to self-report for fear of letting down teammates or not playing up to their multi-million-dollar contracts (Benton, 2017). Additionally, the lack of fully guaranteed contracts in the NFL compared to other American professional sports leagues puts undue pressure on football players to potentially choose between job security and long-term health (Volin, 2016). This dichotomous space of risk and reward is central to the ever-present hegemonic masculine ideology that maintains a grasp on football unlike any other sport, and media is in a position of social responsibility versus corporate partners to provide a space for public discourse and debate about the long-term sustainability of America's sport. Additionally, players who choose to take control of their health should not be chastised, especially since they are the ones putting their bodies—and brains—on the line.

In this context, media play a key role in the dissemination of information, especially to promulgate a cultural shift toward health advocacy on behalf of the players (Sanderson et al., 2016). Social media offers a new avenue for journalists and athletes to provide perspective on head injuries. With the mass following afforded to players via social media platforms, players could influence their social circles to make better decisions. Specifically, when players use the power of social media to share their story, they add to the narrative about traumatic brain injuries. For example, in response to Adams's statement that the football field would be a perfect place to die, Green Bay Packers tight end and ten-year NFL veteran Martellus Bennett tweeted a pair of rebuttals. First, "I hope All [sic] these young cats that are willing to die for the game of football find a higher purpose in life." Bennett followed that with "Look football is great but I ain't dying for this shit. Lol." Add their stories to the voice of journalists who are keeping tabs on changes made in the medical field and other related advancements, and there is an opportunity to keep this issue at the forefront.

With the audience reach a television network can command during a single game, media's responsibility is to not only analyze and critique the game but also to impart knowledge to their viewers. Despite a bifurcation across traditional or digital platforms to a detriment of print, media outlets still have a wealth of options at their disposal. Using these means to produce informative, insightful advertisements or commentary may provide athletes with alternative ways to express their thoughts and concerns. As Oates (2017) explained, "professional football is arguably *the* key symbolic space in the contemporary United States for working through anxieties, contradictions, and hierarchies of dominant masculinities" (p. 7), and media has an opportunity to engage in deep, cultural discussions to work through that symbolic space of masculinity.

The next chapter introduces Mike Webster as a microcosm of masculinity in American football and the long-term effect of adhering to that dominant norm. Additionally, it traces the medical and linguistic history of chronic traumatic encephalopathy from its punch-drunk origin in boxing to its current acronym. Finally, the history of the NFL's MTBI Committee helps position how the league originally responded to brain injuries. This understanding is significant before analyzing how media framed CTE in sport, primarily in football, as a public health concern (Guskiewicz et al., 2005; McCrea et al., 2003; Rabinovici, 2017; Stern et al., 2011).

FOUR

From Punch-Drunk to CTE

The Evolution of a Brain Disease

Mike Webster exemplified the play-through-pain mentality that has fueled football hegemonic masculine ideals for more than a century. More importantly, he exemplified the risk and long-term consequences upheld through adherence to that ideal. Webster played seventeen NFL seasons with the Pittsburgh Steelers and Kansas City Chiefs from 1974 to 1990. After a standout college career at the University of Wisconsin, Webster played 245 career NFL games and started 150 consecutive games as a center. He was part of four Steelers teams to win a Super Bowl (1975, 1976, 1979, 1980). During that illustrious run and beyond, Webster anchored the offensive line, earned seven All-Pro awards, played on nine Pro Bowl teams, and earned the nickname "Iron Mike" both for his durability and his style of play. Arguably the most decorated player in NFL history at his position, Webster was a harbinger both on the field and after his playing career.

For all of Webster's on-field accomplishments, he was inducted into the Pro Football Hall of Fame in Canton, Ohio, on July 26, 1997. He was the seventh player from Pittsburgh's "Steel Curtain" Super Bowl dynasty and the fourteenth of now twenty-one Steelers players to receive the sport's highest honor of immortal enshrinement. Quarterback Terry Bradshaw, who was inducted in 1989, introduced Webster at the 1997 ceremony. They shared the most intimate bond two players can have on the football field, which Bradshaw famously intimated during his own introduction speech: "What I wouldn't give right now to put my hands under Mike Webster's butt just one more time" (Rollow, 1989). At the end of Webster's introduction, Bradshaw removed a football from under the podium, handed it to Webster, and received one final snap in a poignant exchange between center and quarterback.

Webster's twenty-one-minute speech might be the most telling or provocative that, twenty years later, resonates as a moment of foreshadowing that could not have been more eloquently scripted. Webster notably struggled to link disparate parts of his life but had moments of clarity in his speech that offered a glimpse of the struggles he dealt with after his playing career. After thanking family, friends, teammates, and talking about the love of the game, Webster provided a simple truism about playing football for more than half his life.

> It's painful to play football, obviously. It's not fun out there being two-a-day drills in the heat of the summer, banging heads. It's not a natural thing. Football is kind of rare in that it tests you mentally, physically, and emotionally in so many ways. And you know the worst part about that is that it's on film.

Two specific references resonate from this short statement. First, Webster described a physical toll that is clear for anyone who can see the game in person or on film, but it is the repeated act of "banging heads" over any other repetition performed in practice where Webster focused his attention. Webster's playing style at center, where the first point of contact always occurs in football, has been described repeatedly as leading with his head to gain leverage against a defensive lineman. It also led a doctor to ask about excessive scar tissue in Webster's head and whether it was related to a car crash (Mills, 1997).

Second, Webster identified the pain associated with football as rare and unnatural, and published research has validated that his position as an offensive lineman can lead to a life of opioid use and misuse during a playing career to manage injury-related pain (Cottler et al., 2011). Webster became an iconic image at that rare and painful intersection. Ironically, it was in the moment of celebrating the pinnacle of his football achievements that Webster discussed his struggles in a candid and sincere way that highlighted why players continue to play a game despite the daily reminders of its physical, mental, and emotional distress. This idea of pain and overcoming it to achieve football success, as discussed in the previous chapter, is grounded in NFL lore (Butterworth, 2014; Rodgers, 2014). Thus, football as a cultural and social phenomenon debunks civility in sport and replaces it with celebrations of a smash-mouth game.

In the weeks leading to Webster's Hall induction, media reports circulated about his post-NFL career that left him destitute, homeless, addicted to painkillers, and demented as well as divorced and financially broke in just seven years after his playing career. Webster was diagnosed with brain damage in 1999 and showed similar effects of a punch-drunk boxer (Pierson, 2002). Sadly, less than three years later, Webster died September 24, 2002, from a reported heart attack. However, "the real story was far more complicated and sobering" (Cantu and Hyman, 2012, p. 89) for the fifty-year-old football icon.

In life and death, media depicted Webster as a broken-down hero for one of the NFL's most storied franchises and as a case study for the long-term effects that football can have on the body and mind. Pasquarelli (1997) explained the day after Webster's speech that "his soul, if it could be examined, likely would appear to have taken a hit of buckshot" (p. 4E). Webster's mind and soul were dedicated to football. His relentless pursuit of excellence with each repetition in practice and every snap in games reflects on the oddity of his chosen sport, one that requires repeating often minute details from hand position on the ground to angles to leverage that must be attained by every player on the field to make an offense successful (Stade, 1966). Reflecting again on Webster's enshrinement speech, he highlighted a team-first mentality, and that "the greatest thing that's happened to me in my experience in professional football is to have the opportunity to work with people with a common goal and with the same purpose and to sacrifice." Pierson (2002) wrote the day after Webster's death, "For as much as he put into football, Mike Webster wouldn't want to hear that it was the game that killed him" (para. 1). Webster's legacy has shifted from his playing career to his afterlife role as an unexpected poster child for a link between brain trauma and the NFL. However, before outlining how the NFL reached the public ire connected to brain injuries, it is necessary to define CTE and trace its history, which was not extensive in volume prior to Webster but nearly predates the NFL's creation in 1922.

FROM PUNCH-DRUNK TO CTE IN BOXING

CTE is understood as a neurodegenerative condition caused by repeated head trauma (Mez et al, 2017). It is unique from other neurological disorders because of its progressive tauopathy that shows signs much later than when repetitive head injuries likely occurred (Gavett, Stern, Cantu, Nowinski, & McKee, 2010; McKee et al., 2009), many of which may have gone unnoticed by anyone other than the individual who suffered the injury. These injuries can occur in a range of ways from falling on the ground to an automobile accident. The most documented injuries associated with CTE are concussive and sub-concussive head trauma related to contact sports such as boxing, football, hockey, mixed martial arts (MMA), rugby, and wrestling. However, other sports where head trauma can occur, including baseball, soccer, and lacrosse, have documented cases of CTE.

CTE can only be definitively diagnosed postmortem and mirrors many of the symptoms linked to other neurodegenerative conditions (e.g., Alzheimer's, ALS, dementia, Parkinson's) but has a clearly distinct tauopathy (McKee et al., 2016). The challenge for "seeing" CTE is that any outward signs might mimic these other diseases, which have long been associated with their respective symptoms through medically verified research of living patients. Thus, these diseases were perhaps afforded more legitimacy regarding the public being able to identify with the diseases and their subsequent progressions. A few institutes drive most of the CTE-centered research. The Brain Injury Research Institute (BIRI) was founded in 2002 by Omalu, Julian Bailes, and Robert Fitzsimmons. The CTE Center is an independent collection of researchers affiliated with the Alzheimer's Disease Center at Boston University. Ann McKee is the director of this brain bank that studies brains often donated by families of athletes who died and were suspected to have suffered repetitive head injuries. Additionally, a group of researchers at the University of California at Los Angeles (UCLA) patented FDDNP, a chemical marker that claims to identify tau tangles in the brains of living individuals with the assistance of a PET scan but still requires postmortem confirmation (Omalu et al., 2018). With each new batch of brains, tau proteins, and researchers, the desire and funding opportunities to study CTE continue to explode with headline-grabbing statistics, but questions remain about the validity of these findings.

As football has dominated the research and media rhetoric, the origin—and originality or lack thereof—of chronic traumatic encephalopathy is often lost in the public domain, including a few iterative name changes in the twentieth century. Science literature credits Harrison Martland with the seminal research linking blows to the head through repetitive punching in boxing to long-term head trauma resulting in neurological abnormalities ranging from mild to severe. Martland (1928) examined twenty-three boxers and described a condition as "punch drunk" in which "there is a very definite brain injury due to single or repeated blows on the head or jaw which cause multiple concussion hemorrhages in the deeper portions of the cerebrum" that evolve into a "degenerative progressive lesion" (p. 1103). Martland linked punch-drunk as a cause of Parkinsonian syndrome.

The 1930s witnessed two new medical labels to advance Martland's research and evolve punch-drunk into more clinical terms. Traumatic encephalopathy (Parker, 1934) and dementia pugilistica (Millspaugh, 1937) emerged after each study examined pugilists, which later shifted linguistically to the more commonly known term boxer. Parker (1934) worked at the Mayo Clinic in Minnesota and observed three boxers who were admitted between 1923 and 1934. After assessing these three cases, Parker offered that each boxer had suffered from brain injury that varied in longevity of impact and that agreement was only available by a "suggestion of diffuse or scattered lesions of the brain affecting different systems" (p. 28). He noted a lack of pathological insight since a postmortem diagnosis was not an option. Additionally, Parker only used traumatic encephalopathy once in the entire paper, so it did not advance the terminology beyond offering it as an alternative term to Martland's punch-drunk.

Millspaugh (1937) advanced "punch-drunk" to "dementia pugilistica." Like Parker, one noticeable limitation is that the term is only used once in the article beyond the title. Millspaugh spoke with U.S. Navy medical doctors who often examined boxers and observed fights. Their observations were considered valid since the NCAA used the naval boxing guidelines for assessing fighters before matches. Yes, the NCAA had boxing as a sanctioned sport until 1960 (Wallenfeldt, 1994). That year, University of Wisconsin boxer Charlie Mohr suffered a brain hemorrhage following his final fight at the NCAA tournament and died eight days later (Kane, 1960). Millspaugh's research, however, was later described as "clinically inaccurate" (Johnson, 1969, p. 45; Unterharnscheidt & Taylor-Unterharnscheidt, 2003, p. 294) for its link to dementia and limitation to naval researchers examining semiprofessional fighters. The findings advanced a new name for repeated head trauma but did little else except to offer a linkage in his one reference to dementia pugilistica that its "etiology . . . is trauma" (p. 299) from repetitive and frequent injuries to the head.

Dementia pugilistica has a problematic, yet long-standing, history. Martland never mentioned dementia pugilistica in his seminal publication. However, he has been mistakenly credited with the term to describe the trauma boxers exhibited in his study (Levin & Bhardwaj, 2014; Omalu, Fitzsimmons, Hammers, & Bailes, 2010; Patricios & Kemp, 2014). In other published research, dementia pugilistica is attributed to secondary sources (Concannon et al., 2014; Mendez, 1995) or assumed as public knowledge with no citation (Gavett et al., 2010; Gilbert & Johnson, 2011; Merz, Van Patten, & Lace, 2017; Saffary et al., 2012; Wortzel, 2014). This unassociated past is interesting considering it is the medical terminology that would describe the long-term effects of repetitive head trauma in boxers for nearly seventy years during a slow evolution toward CTE.

As far as the research for this book could identity, it was more than a decade until Critchley (1949) provided the first known reference to "chronic traumatic encephalopathy" that advanced punch-drunkenness to a progressive medical issue with lasting neurological and psychological concerns. He provided an extensive literature review of chronic issues specific to brain trauma in boxing and explained "the course of this disorder (CTE) is unusual, because . . . it is progressive despite the cessation of the causative trauma" (Critchley, 1949, p. 134). Additionally, he identified a significant lapse in time between when a boxer first competed in the sport and when the psychological and neurological abnormalities began to show. Thus, CTE remained hidden from any outward visible symptoms until long-term effects hindered patients, sometimes for the remainder of their life.

Eight years later, Critchley (1957) advanced the conversation and terminology. First, he provided greater detail about the spectacle of boxing's acute knock-out in its "deliberate and violent production" (p. 357) that parallels football by its "tension inherent . . . in its violence . . . but without becoming so destructive" (Oriard, 2014a, p. 121) as to keep fans from watching or limit participation. Critchley traced the historic terminological shift from punch-drunk caused by an apparent need to "introduce a more esoteric and less offensive expression" (Critchley, 1957, p. 358) that might validate findings connected to the impact of repetitive head trauma in boxing. Based on his research examining sixty-nine cases of boxers, Critchley combined terms from his previously published research into "chronic progressive traumatic encephalopathy" (p. 359) that he claimed was irreversible and steadily advancing. Over time the language for the condition reverted to chronic traumatic encephalopathy.

The 1960s were significant for boxing both in mediated construction of some of the sport's greatest fighters but also for careers later marred by the long-term effects of brain trauma (Solomon, 2018). That decade concluded with two important medical studies. Roberts (1969) published a book that detailed traumatic encephalopathy in British boxers. He concluded that 17 percent of 224 boxers he examined exhibited some form of the disease, with a 50 percent rate for boxers over the age of fifty with more than 150 career fights. Additionally, Johnson (1969) examined seventeen ex-boxers and determined that sixteen had traumatic encephalopathy but only half were progressive. The remaining eight were stationary. Therefore, it made more sense, according to these two studies, to examine for CTE and attempt to differentiate between progressive and stationary (Johnson, 1969; Roberts, 1969).

Neuroscientists began studying brains of ex-boxers beyond the neurological tests administered to living patients. As noted in previous studies, a postmortem examination of the brain could provide telling differences between CTE and other neurodegenerative conditions. Corsellis et al. (1973) produced a significant study of fifteen brains of retired boxers who died over a sixteen-year span and whose brains were collected for examination. As noted from the article's outset, the study was interested in identifying abnormalities in these brains compared to other demented conditions such as Alzheimer's. The authors noted that Alzheimer's patients "virtually always" (p. 296) have neurofibrillary tangles accompanied by senile plagues as consistent signs of the degenerative condition. In their study, the brains of boxers indicated an abundance of tangles with sparse—if any—senile plaques. In their opinion, this was a clear sign of the impact of repeated head trauma as "precipitating, if not causal, agents" (p. 297) for this curious scientific finding. Advances in testing technology led to a study by Roberts, Allsop, and Bruton (1990) that reexamined fourteen of the fifteen brains in the Corsellis et al. study, plus six more, and compared them to twenty brains confirmed with Alzheimer's and twenty age-matched controls. Their examination found extensive similarities to Alzheimer's in the identifying markers previously linked to CTE, which challenged the uniqueness of CTE and raised questions of whether CTE was pathologically or progressively different (Iverson, Keene, Perry, & Castellani, 2018; Randolph, 2018; Solomon, 2018). Regardless, nearly thirty years after Roberts et al., these similar abnormalities sent CTE into the popular press and American lexicon (Randolph, 2014).

Boxing remained the primary focus for CTE research and repetitive head trauma in sport throughout the twentieth century. Neuropsychological tests advanced Critchley's hypothesis of a correlation between the neurological and psychological effects in boxers. Casson et al. (1984) examined eighteen active and retired boxers and performed a battery of neuropsychological tests. They concluded that 87 percent of the fighters in their study had various forms of brain damage and that findings from CT scans "should not be dismissed as a normal variant but should be considered a sign of encephalopathy" (p. 2566). Mendez (1995) offered three stages of the clinical manifestation that characterizes CTE. First, changes in motor skills and personality were visible, including increased irritability and aggression. Second, definitive slowing of cognition was evident in loss of memory and slowed processing of information. Mendez defined the final stage as dementia pugilistica that affected thought and speech daily. Despite advanced understanding of long-term impacts of head injuries, Mendez (1995) reminded that boxing's outcome was intended "to inflict brain trauma on the opponent" (p. 257) and thus changes in rules or equipment could only reduce the significance of the trauma but not eliminate it from the sport.

Boxing provided a longer history of hegemonic masculinity than American football that traced back centuries (Scott, 2017). However, since its roots were not American, U.S. media focused on prize fights, but the sport's scheduling did not lend itself to the level of media attention afforded to football. Ultimately, the long-term cognitive effects rampant in boxing challenged hegemonic masculinity because of "the brutalizing experience which is blatantly savage and destructive, resulting in acute and chronic injuries, mostly to the eyes and brain, and sometimes causing massive hemorrhaging and even death" (Hargreaves, 1997, p. 34). Boxing still maintains a masculine ideology, but in American sports popularity, boxing rarely moved the mediated needle like it did during its heyday in the 1980s.

CONCUSSIONS AND FOOTBALL

While boxing suffered from decades of studies that connected the sport to long-term and debilitating cognitive effects, football was more often connected to concussions, which were considered isolated and singular events. Additionally, the intent of boxing was to inflict direct contact to the head with a knockout as the ultimate achievement. Football provided a different type of contact sport where collisions were expected but could occur through indirect and unexpected hits on the field that produced significant brain injuries. As early as the Harvard study in 1905, concussions were taken lightly by the players and would not serve as a rationale to not compete for the team. Therefore, concussions in football were not a new revelation. The new terrain for concussions started around the 1960s. The challenges included a need for consistent measures for diagnosis, evaluation, and treatment (Buckley, 1988; Gerberich, Priest, Boen, Straub, & Maxwell, 1983; Yarnell & Lynch, 1970). Loss of consciousness and amnesia were considered as visible signs related to concussions but were not required for a concussion diagnosis (Guskiewicz, 2001).

Return-to-play (RTP) guidelines were first established in 1986 by Robert Cantu. Three grades (mild, moderate, and severe) were offered with the most severe including loss of consciousness of more than five minutes with post-traumatic amnesia lasting longer than twenty-four hours. The suggested time away from contact sports was a minimum of one month with the individual being asymptomatic for one week beyond that initial month (Cantu, 1986). A mild concussion (grade 1) was the most common and most difficult to interpret, but an athlete could return if asymptomatic for one week. That period extended to two weeks after a second concussion and called for an athlete to sit for the remainder of a season after a third concussion (Cantu, 1986). These RTP guidelines were intended for all sports, but the connection between concussions and football dominated media coverage and academic research.

Concussions earned the NFL a significant level of media attention beginning in 1992. In a span of less than two years, wide receiver Al Toon and running back Merril Hoge retired due to post-concussion symptoms, and quarterbacks Troy Aikman and Steve Young suffered concussions that resulted in significant memory loss (Heinze & Lu, 2017; Siegler & Wesley, 2016; Smith, 2013; Solomon, 2018). The NFL followed these well-publicized injuries with a tactical maneuver akin to Big Tobacco. Heinze and Lu (2017) identified this strategy as decoupling, which was an organizational strategy utilized to dismiss medical findings and avoid responsibility by implementing symbolic practices that produced no substantive results.

In 1994, commissioner Paul Tagliabue created the Mild Traumatic Brain Injury (MTBI) Committee to study the impact of head injuries. However, it was the equivalent of a knee-jerk reaction to media inquiries amid a league cover-up (Fainaru-Wada & Fainaru, 2013). Tagliabue had a somewhat contentious relationship with media. Just prior to the league's announced MTBI Committee (though it was initially referred to as a league subcommittee), Tagliabue participated in a unique panel at a New

York City YMCA titled "Sports Commissioners Tackle the Future of Major League Sports." This panel included Tagliabue, alongside fellow commissioners David Stern from the National Basketball Association and Gary Bettman of the National Hockey League. Pulitzer Prize–winning journalist David Halberstam moderated the question-and-answer session. The back-and-forth between Halberstam and Tagliabue was reported as combative and annoying, especially when Halberstam shifted the conversation from player contract and labor disputes to concussions and player safety (Fainaru-Wada & Fainaru, 2013; Vescey, 1994).

It was during this panel in December 1994 that Tagliabue dismissed concussions as a "pack journalism issue" (Edelson, 2014; Fainaru-Wada & Fainaru, 2013). Instead, the league's initial research revealed a "relatively small" amount of concussions in the NFL, according to Greg Aiello, the NFL director of communication. Thus, instead of brain injuries as a growing league concern, Tagliabue said the problem was a "journalist issue" (Dahlberg, 2017; Powell, 2017). At the time of Tagliabue's comments, which he confirmed and apologized for in an interview on the *Talk of Fame Sports Network* in 2017 while promoting his unsuccessful campaign for election to the Pro Football Hall of Fame, concussions were starting to garner headlines.

Nine years after the committee formed, it published the first of what mainstream media and scientific journals incorrectly identified as a thirteen-part series on concussions in the medical journal *Neurosurgery* beginning in 2003. Instead, research for this book identified that it was a fourteen-part series with each article beginning with a consistently named title, "Concussion in professional football." Thus, anytime the MTBI Committee studies are mentioned henceforth in this book, it will be referred to as fourteen parts. One other point of concern regarding where the studies were published was that the journal's editor, Michael Apuzzo, was a consultant with the New York Giants.

Tagliabue wrote a guest editorial in the same issue as the first published study. He noted, "we realized that there were many more questions than answers" (Tagliabue, 2003, p. 796) but that research was needed to examine and hopefully better understand concussions in football. Tagliabue appointed Elliot Pellman, who was a rheumatologist and New York Jets team doctor, to chair the MTBI Committee. Pellman was lead author for nine of the fourteen articles published in *Neurosurgery*. The first study used video from television broadcasts between 1996 and 2001 to examine 182 head injuries sustained during NFL games. The reconstructed videos analyzed head impact velocity and changes in velocity and determined "a striking observation" (Pellman, Viano, Tucker, Casson, & Waeckerle, 2003, p. 808) in which players sustained "exceptionally high velocities and accelerations and long duration" (p. 808) from the injuries included in their study of concussions. The findings called for better helmet technology and fines for violators of new rules designed to reduce targeting the head during games.

Around the same time as the MTBI Committee's first published report, surveys of high school and college football players gathered through questionnaires sent to athletic trainers identified greater risk of concussion recurrence following a first concussion that produced lower test scores compared to baseline numbers for cognitive impairment and balance problems immediately following a concussion. These studies indicated symptoms lasting up to seven days following a concussion (Guskiewicz et al., 2003; Guskiewicz, Weaver, Padua, & Garrett, 2000; McCrea et al., 2003). The same cohort of scientists advanced this research through a survey of 2,552 retired professional football players. The findings identified that players with a history of concussions were at greater risk for lifelong depression and memory loss as well as early onset of dementia (Guskiewicz et al., 2005; Guskiewicz et al., 2007).

These findings were challenged by the MTBI Committee who provided contrary information. Nowinski (2007) noted the "most controversial paper" (p. 93) was the fourth publication in the fourteen-part series. This six-year study used information from standardized reports provided by NFL team physicians regarding 887 concussions across 650 players. Nearly one-fourth of players (n = 161, 24.8 percent) experienced a repeat concussion, and 51 players (7.8 percent) suffered three or more concussions. Their findings indicated 57.5 percent of players returned to play within one day after a second concussion (Pellman et al., 2004). The problematic findings challenged that players were not susceptible to a repeat concussion within the seven- to ten-day window identified by Guskiewicz et al.'s study of college football players, thus minimizing any concern for a player's vulnerability to a secondary injury that could have longer cognitive effects (Pellman et al., 2004).

Exposés such as *League of Denial* have intricately detailed how the NFL championed faulty research (Fainaru-Wada & Fainaru, 2013). The NFL's creation and use of the MTBI Committee appeared to have many parallels to the TIRC and Big Tobacco, which further perpetuated a perceived connection between these two industries and their attempt to tamp down talk of environmental hazards. This raised serious ethical questions regarding ties between MTBI Committee members with the NFL and concern regarding the conflicts of interest present when it came time to publish the scientific results. In the fourteen-part, peer-reviewed academic papers in *Neurosurgery*, the committee stated repeatedly it relied upon complete data provided by team medical staff from 1996 through 2001 that was mandated by then NFL-commissioner Tagliabue and coded to maintain player anonymity (Pellman, Viano, Casson, Arfken, & Feuer, 2005).

Schwarz et al. (2016) identified through "confidential peer-review documents, the committee wrote that 'all N.F.L. teams participated' and that 'all players were therefore part of the study'" (para. 26). However, *The New York Times* investigation contradicted these statements by looking at publicly available injury databases and noted that most teams had failed to document each players' injuries, with several teams (such as the Dallas Cowboys and San Francisco 49ers) having no concussions listed for years at a time, which was clearly not the case when looking at public injury data (Schwarz et al., 2016). Even after repeated academic reviewers pointed out serious flaws with the conflict of interest present in the studies, the journal ignored these comments and moved forward with publishing the results. One anonymous reviewer even wrote "many of the management of concussion suggestions are inappropriate and not founded on facts" (Schwarz et al., 2016, p. 7). Big Tobacco once had a playbook—which served as a master plan and script that directed the behavior of industry executives, lobbyists, lawyers, and scientists—that emphasized the "not proven" rhetoric to bring public doubt to the science that already existed (Brownell & Warner, 2009; Paolini, 2019). This playbook was eerily like the one used by the NFL.

The MTBI Committee published its research at a rapid rate. In the fifteen months between October 2003 and February 2005, the first eight articles were published and gained widespread media attention. This started to promote the NFL's desired narrative that the league was proactive and working toward better understanding concussions in football. It was revealed roughly a decade after these published reports that in 1997 the NFL hired lawyer Dorothy Mitchell, who previously defended the Tobacco Institute, to provide legal counsel to the MTBI Committee. Mitchell's efforts were credited with providing significant momentum behind the initial MTBI research (Fainaru-Wada & Fainaru, 2013; Schwartz et al., 2016). The NFL was a self-described leader in the fight against concussions (and potentially long-term brain injuries). However, in an ironic twist, *Neurosurgery*, the same journal that promoted the NFL propaganda written by the MTBI Committee, published an article in July 2005 that provided the beginning of scientific research that challenged the league narrative and resurrected CTE from a decades-long hiatus in medical journal lexicon (Randolph, 2018).

ADVOCATE FOR THE DEAD

Bennet Omalu is a Nigerian-born pathologist who moved to the United States in 1994 to pursue a medical career. Omalu spent his first year at the University of Washington as a visiting/research scholar in the department of epidemiology. A four-year residency in pathology followed at Harlem Hospital Center in New York City. Then in 1999, he moved to Pittsburgh and completed a one-year fellowship in forensic pathology at the Allegheny County Coroner's Office and a two-year fellowship in neuropathology at the University of Pittsburgh Medical Center. Between 2002 and 2005, Omalu received board certifications in anatomic pathology, clinical pathology, forensic pathology, and neuropathology.

During his formative years in Pittsburgh, Omalu received some media exposure, primarily as a medical expert in several court cases followed by local media. A Lexis-Nexis search for his name connected him to five stories between 2004 and 2005. In 2004, he testified in a manslaughter trial of a midwife charged in an infant's death. Later that year, Omalu testified in another manslaughter case stemming from a Pennsylvania diner dispute. In 2005, Omalu was quoted in three articles. First, Omalu defended then–Allegheny County coroner Cyril Wecht in an article that raised conflict-of-interest questions. Wecht conducted private autopsies for surrounding counties where Omalu helped after hours (Conti, 2005). Second, Omalu testified about an infant death from Shaken Baby Syndrome (Foreman, 2005). Third, Omalu was connected for the first time to the NFL and CTE. Omalu defended his autopsy findings that former Steelers offensive lineman Terry Long, who died from drinking antifreeze, had CTE, and that the "repetitive and cumulative effect" of blows to the head from football was the cause (Greenwood, 2005, para. 9).

It was prior to Omalu's initial media exposure that he unknowingly started a journey that would elevate him and CTE to global notoriety. That journey began on September 28, 2002, when Omalu arrived for work at the coroner's office and Webster's body awaited him four days after his death. Fainaru-Wada and Fainaru (2013) dubbed that day as "one of the most significant dates in the history of American sports. You won't find it in the record books" (p. 2). The initial death certificate listed post-concussion syndrome as contributing to the cause of death. Omalu saved Webster's brain despite its initial normal appearance. Omalu returned to Webster's brain two weeks later for further examination that identified Webster as a "victim" of football because his "brain revealed the tissue substrates of gridiron dementia or football-induced chronic traumatic encephalopathy" (Omalu, 2008, p. 89). However, it would be three years before the medical world and media would reunite around Webster's death, his brain, and football.

The summer of 2005 proved to be the launching point for Omalu's career and the long-term union between CTE and the NFL, but Omalu predicted the impact his research would have in a 2004 abstract for a presentation at the annual meeting for the American Association of Neuropathologists. In that abstract, which was published in the *Journal of Neuropathology & Experimental Neurology*, Omalu (2004) wrote that the NFL's MTBI Committee had not correctly focused on the effects of "repeated concussion brain injury" (p. 535) in football players for its first published studies beginning in 2003. The abstract concluded with:

> this report constitutes a forensic epidemiological sentinel case that may justify the need for a forensic autopsy registry for retired NFL players for comprehensive tissue diagnosis and generation of empirical data on the association of professional football and long term neurodegeneration (p. 535).

While this presentation preceded his well-publicized published report of Webster's brain by one year, Omalu seemed to know the importance of these findings but that significantly more data would be necessary to offer any long-term understanding.

Omalu et al. (2005) published the first documented case of CTE in a football player. The authors noted "this case study by itself cannot confirm a causal link between professional football and CTE" (p. 132) and called for more empirical research to determine if football causes CTE. Just one month prior to publishing Webster's seminal case, Long died on June 7. A teammate of Webster's for five years, Long played eight seasons in Pittsburgh from 1984 to 1991. Long was examined by Omalu and determined to have signs of CTE that were distinct from Webster (Omalu et al., 2006). The cause of death was clear, but the causal link that drove Long to suicide was determined by Omalu as beyond his control. In each of these cases, Omalu (2008) explained his role as a forensic pathologist "as advocates for the dead. We defend and speak for the dead" (p. 88) in hope of applying that knowledge to save lives.

Omalu is often credited with diagnosing the first case of CTE in an NFL player, but he did not "discover" CTE as was widely misrepresented in media and other published reports. The history of CTE's discovery is thoroughly and historically traced in this chapter. Regardless, Omalu was belittled in correspondence to his research by three members of the MTBI Committee who called for his published studies to be retracted or substantially revised because of "speculative" findings. Ironically, given the NFL's questionable published reports, the authors wrote, "we think full disclosure of all facts by all parties is necessary for a full and open 'scholarly discussion and understanding' regarding this important matter" (Casson, Pellman, & Viano, 2006, p. E1152). Since Omalu et al.'s initial findings, CTE has risen to a level of public debate fueled by a media storm, thousands of medical journal articles, and calls for the NFL to engage in that same full and open discussion suggested by members of its own committee. Understanding of CTE's cause and long-term impact on sport remains muddied because of scientific debates between isolated cases and diagnoses versus scientifically verifiable data and the use of those isolated studies by media (Ban, Madden, Bailes, Batjer, & Lonser, 2016).

THE NFL'S RESPONSE

The composition of the MTBI Committee and limited credentials of some of its members raised substantial concerns because of direct connections to the league or teams that provided what was perceived as biased and unreliably produced findings (Fainaru-Wada & Fainaru, 2013). Additionally, ethical questions regarding medical professionals paying professional sports teams millions of dollars to be an "official" team doctor for marketing purposes challenge the validity of information provided by the MTBI Committee studies (Nowinski, 2007; Pennington, 2004). Pellman served as chairman from 1994 until 2005 when a *New York Times* article claimed he exaggerated his resume, including misrepresenting where he earned his medical degree. He attended medical school in Mexico, not State University New York at Stony Brook as he claimed, which is where he earned a degree after a one-year residency. Interestingly, Pellman's inflated credentials were discovered while he served as a medical adviser to Major League Baseball during congressional hearings on steroids (Wilson, 2005). Pellman remained as a member of the MTBI Committee until the NFL disbanded it in 2010 amid pressure from Congress. Commissioner Goodell replaced the MTBI Committee with the newly formed Head, Neck, and Spine (HNS) Committee and named Hunt Batjer and Richard Ellenbogen as co-chairs. Batjer was chair of neurological surgery at Northwestern University, and Ellenbogen was chair of neurological surgery at the University of Washington (Ellenbogen, Berger, & Batjer, 2010). Pellman's affiliation with the NFL officially ended in 2016 when he retired as a league medical adviser on the recommendation of commissioner Goodell (Seifert, 2016a).

While still members of the MTBI Committee, Pellman and Viano (2006) published a study (not one of the fourteen in *Neurosurgery*) that examined 787 cases (from 1,913 games) of game-related mild traumatic brain injuries and noted that 56.5 percent of players who suffered a concussion during an NFL game returned to play in the same game. Based on these findings, the authors noted that "it can be concluded that mild TBIs in professional football *are not serious injuries*" (Pellman & Viano, 2006, p. 6, emphasis added). Nowinski (2007) quoted an anonymous researcher affiliated with the NFL who said the fourteen-part series was "becoming everyone's gospel, and that's dangerous" (p. 92) because of the questionable data.

The gospel publications were at least a recognition by the NFL of a recurring problem of concussions and brain injuries in football, albeit not generated by independent, neurological experts. However, the league denied any direct connection between these head injuries and loss of long-term cognitive function (Asplund & Best, 2015; Goldberg, 2013; Heiner, 2008). Despite these denials, the NFL started a strategic funding campaign that followed an important court case. A 2006 ruling by the

Fourth Circuit Court of Appeals awarded disability status posthumously to Webster "holding that he was mentally incapacitated to a point of suffering 'total and permanent disability as a result of football'" (Heiner, 2008, p. 257, citing *Jani v. Bert Bell/Pete Rozell Players Ret. Plan*).

In 2007, the NFL announced for the first time a league-wide concussion management plan to assess when a player should return to game action (Heiner, 2008) and that a player could not return on the same day if he lost consciousness (Neale, 2009). When the league announced the initial concussion policy, it continued to deny any connection between properly treated concussions and long-term effects (Kain, 2009). Additionally, in 2007, the NFL approved $17 million in funding to assist former players with medical support services ("Chronology of," 2017). While statistical data indicated a significant rise in concussions, Harrison (2014) explained the dilemma well since "the concussion crisis is commonly framed as a battle over evidence and a need for new technical solutions" (p. 823). Concussions were clearly an issue in football, but how they were diagnosed, reported, monitored, and addressed was still of critical concern both for the safety of athletes and clarity of medical guidelines.

Beyond the NFL, concussions in football reached an initial crisis level and legislative intervention in 2009, three years after thirteen-year-old Zackery Lystedt incurred "significant neurological injury and residual disabilities that affect almost every activity of daily life" (Adler & Herring, 2011, p. S468). Lystedt suffered a head injury during a middle school football game, but he returned to play without any assessment from a medically trained professional and collapsed after making the last tackle of the game. Lystedt survived following emergency brain surgery, but his story received significant attention and his injuries confined him to a wheelchair (Bernstein, 2012). Lystedt was not the first football player to suffer a serious head injury, but his name was forever associated with legal changes geared toward safety directly connected to concussions. On May 14, 2009, Washington governor Christine Gregoire signed the Zackery Lystedt Law aimed to educate coaches, players, and medical staff of the dangers of head injuries and mandated that a player who suffered a head injury was not to return to the field until given medical clearance. By 2014, all fifty states and the District of Columbia signed similar legislation (Adler & Herring, 2011; Albano, Adler, Herring, & Asif, 2016; Bernstein, 2012).

On December 2, 2009, the NFL announced an updated concussion policy that barred a player from returning to a game or practice on the same day he suffered a concussion and outlined more specific return-to-play guidelines. Schwarz (2009) reported "symptoms that require immediate removal include amnesia, poor balance, and an abnormal neurological examination" (p. A3) but that players with dizziness or headaches could return to play if the symptoms were not persistent. Additionally, these changes contradicted the findings and recommendations from the NFL's published findings in *Neurosurgery*. Over the next seven years, the NFL continued to tweak the league's concussion protocol and announced a "Play Smart. Play Safe." initiative in 2016 with four goals: protecting players, advanced technology, medical research, and sharing progress. The NFL press release identified the league had implemented forty-two rule changes since 2002 for player protection, education, better methods of practice, and stronger medical protocols that included harsh penalties for any team that failed to enforce the NFL Game Day Concussion Protocol ("NFL announces," 2016).

AVAILABILITY CASCADE, CTE, AND THE NFL

As concussions gained significant traction during the 2000s, it was somewhere between 2007 and 2009 when CTE started to make its way into medical and public discourse before a cascade of published scientific research and media reports followed beginning in 2010. A few significant moments contributed to this surge. First, the suicide of former NFL player Andre Waters in 2006 and the murder committed by professional wrestler Chris Benoit in 2007 of his wife and son before killing himself started to circulate beyond the isolated cases of Webster and Long. Second, Omalu et al. (2006) published a second case of CTE diagnosed in an American football player. Additionally, Omalu (2008) wrote his first book, *Play Hard, Die Young*, that linked dementia, depression, and death to repetitive brain trauma that he claimed resulted in CTE. Connections were starting to form both in media stories and medical findings between brain trauma, memory loss, and suicide.

Along with Omalu, Chris Nowinski became a strong voice in the public fight for recognition of CTE. A former college football player, professional wrestler, and Harvard Ph.D., Nowinski provided a link between all the key prominent CTE researchers. Nowinski was not a medical professional, but he was passionate about the long-term effects of brain injuries in sport after suffering post-concussion syndrome that forced his retirement from wrestling. He connected with Omalu to examine Waters's brain, which resulted in a CTE diagnosis. In 2007, Nowinski and Robert Cantu formed the Sports Legacy Institute, which was later renamed the Concussion Legacy Foundation. In 2008, their group partnered with the Boston University School of Medicine and the VA and created the Center for the Study of Traumatic Encephalopathy (later renamed the CTE Center). These key moments along with three more highly publicized cases of CTE in deceased NFL players formed the foundation for increased media exposure and a precipitous availability cascade of published scientific research of CTE without empirical merit (Ban et al., 2016; Barr, 2013; Davis, Castellani, & McCrory, 2015; Gaetz, 2017; Kuhn, Yengo-Khan, Kerr, & Zuckerman, 2017; Solomon, 2018).

While these newly formed groups worked with "ground-breaking" research, it must be noted that Wolfson (1938) identified football in connection with traumatic encephalopathy in his published research of varying psychiatric medical links to brain injuries. However, much like the early research on punch-drunk syndrome and dementia pugilistica in boxers, which relied on donated brains after people died, the number of brains showing signs of CTE continued to increase as more professional athletes (mostly American football players) died and donated their brains to science. One overriding concern was—and remains—that biased samples produced questionable research findings that could not be compared to any other available research data (Alosco et al., 2019; Asken & Bauer, 2018; DeKosky, Jaffee, & Bauer, 2018; Mez et al., 2017; Solomon, 2018).

Newspapers around the world started to inundate the public with stories that referenced CTE. Of the news stories used in the research for this book, the number of stories combined across six newspapers between 2006 and 2008 that mentioned CTE totaled only fourteen articles. That number nearly doubled to twenty-six in 2010. It increased nearly four-fold by 2013 to ninety-two articles before it reached a peak in 2016 across the six newspapers with a combined 199 articles. This rapid increase of news exposure paralleled the scientific push for more published research.

Thus, brain injuries reported in connection with football focused on CTE. This created an availability cascade, despite medical limitations and sampling questions, that produced "discursive clashes between emotionally charged representations of CTE as a widespread, urgent health problem and commentary cautioning audiences about the degree of scientific uncertainty surrounding CTE" (Ventresca, 2018, p. 12). Barr (2013) explained the role of media in overlooking data for high-profile cases involving athletes recovering from brain injuries that created a divergence between public perception and medical findings. Reliance on family members for recall of history of brain injuries further neglected necessary empirical data in control groups (Gaetz, 2017) but created tantalizing news stories of family struggles. Solomon and Sills (2014) explained that inflated media coverage and lack of properly controlled sample groups related to CTE was a prime example of how an availability cascade worked to create "social psychological pressures leading individuals to believe, endorse, and perpetuate the biased perception" (p. 27). The cascade of information related to brain injuries, most specific to CTE, has not always passed on accurate information, patterns of diagnosis, or methods for examination and resulted in charges of confusion and misinformation that has been a concern for lack of evidence since the NFL and CTE were connected (Granier et al., 2011; Randolph, 2014). Finkel and Bienick (2018) later noted the risk of falling prey to the availability cascade argument that can cloud how evidence was perceived. However, the cascade of information quickly mounted. Add in a growing number of legal cases involving football—mostly the NFL—connected to brain injuries, and media attention helped fuel a public health crisis (Solomon, 2018).

As a final thought for this chapter, it is helpful to circle back to Webster's Hall of Fame speech. It is unclear what provoked this prescient part of his speech, but it resonated long after his death about why CTE research would be important moving forward for science and football in what must be a collaborative effort.

> You know what, we're in this damn thing together folks. And I'm talking about the things that are going on today that have been ignored for a long period of time, and yeah, we're addressing them now because we have a history of only addressing them when they jump up and bite us in the ass, and not until we do that. But we can change that. We can change, but we're in this together. We gotta care about one another. We gotta care about our kids.

A cultural shift to recognize and take concussions and brain injuries seriously has been a slow, arduous process (Nowinski, 2007). It took decades for the NFL to admit a link between brain injuries suffered while playing football and long-term cognitive effects (e.g., dementia). Right or wrong, the NFL is the standard by which research must guide a shift from "getting your bell rung" to understanding the long-term impact for its former, current, and future players to help those impacted by brain injuries.

The next three chapters turn to the significant analysis provided in this book. They offer insight into how media framed CTE as a disease, as an NFL problem, and ultimately, as a football epidemic to be considered as a public health issue. Before diving into the analysis, the next chapter starts with a basic understanding of the historical purpose of science research and journalism as well as the difficult, yet necessary, relationship between science and media.

FIVE

Mediating Science

The Framing of CTE

Scientific research is said to work toward advancing knowledge, either through cumulative data analysis or theoretical testing (Nelson, 1959). Often collected over time, this information is organized, processed, and analyzed before producing what scientists hope can be verifiable and generalizable information to move knowledge forward. Who and what defines science is debatable, but it is often divided into hard (e.g., natural and physical) versus soft science (e.g., social and behavioral) with varying outcome goals of replicable practices (Hedges, 1987). Regardless of type of scientific study, the outcome of these findings can be linked to economic gain by many powerful organizations (e.g., governmental, hospitals, pharmaceutical companies, universities, sports league) but also for public consumption and awareness (Nelson, 1959).

How scientists deliver their findings offers another level of analysis and critique, both in preparation and presentation, as evident in chapter 2 regarding the framing of tobacco and HIV/AIDS to affect public perception. Researchers like to describe their findings as filling a "gap" in the literature. An existing gap is identified through a systematic and thorough literature review that positions the researcher's knowledge and understanding of what work has been done in a subject discipline (Hart, 1998). Ultimately, a gap provides a quest for new knowledge to an unanswered question. Kearney (2017) explains that "filling a gap requires identification of a problem of some degree of social import" (p. 393). Therefore, a research study should answer a question through an original contribution to a knowledge gap that positions where it fits within the outlined literature review (Hart, 1998). The findings can be large or small because a significant contribution should be measured in quality of the research, not necessarily the size of the contribution or quantity of data or participants (Hart, 1998; Kearney, 2017).

The presentation of findings is significant for positioning a research project within a "gap." Hyland (1996) describes a practice of hedging in scientific writing as a linguistic strategy to support new findings but also avoid redress when challenging previously established data or theory where a gap was identified. This notion of hedging in academic writing is a strategic approach of politeness to avoid redress but allows space to gain recognition in a researcher's academic field that is likely flush with published journal articles that are already considered conceptual, theoretical, and empirical (Myers, 1989). Hedging is more commonly applied to spoken word as a form of negative politeness with the intention to mitigate derogation of another person (Brown & Levinson, 1978; Goffman, 1956; Leech, 2014). The use of hedges in published scientific research establishes "an essential element of argumentation in presenting new claims for ratification and are among the primary features which shape the research article as the principle vehicle for new knowledge" (Hyland, 1996, p. 452). The intent of hedging is strategic and purposeful.

CTE researchers required a similar approach in early published work, especially given the limited number of cases and clear concerns regarding convenience samples, to distinguish CTE from other neurodegenerative brain diseases such as Alzheimer's, amyotrophic lateral sclerosis (ALS or Lou Gehrig's disease), dementia, and Parkinson's. More than a decade after Omalu et al.'s seminal publication, Rabinovici (2017) attempted to synthesize CTE research by identifying advances and gaps in existing CTE findings with a goal of offering future research ideas because "the fundamental questions about the disorder remain unresolved" (p. 339). Thus, his literature review provided an example of hedging in CTE research to politely define a gap in the existing scientific work.

While some scientists might work toward polite forms of redress in identifying new research possibilities to avoid challenging established leaders in a discipline, others utilize the notion of debunking to advance an ideologically opposed idea. The purpose of debunking is an intent to expose some sense of falseness or to discredit someone's reputation. This strategy has been used to debunk perceived myths concerning causes of cancer (Biswas, 2014), transfer of HIV in pools (Nair, 2000), environmental risks (Sandman, 1994), and what percentage of a brain is used by humans (Vreeman & Carroll, 2007), to name a few. As outlined in chapter 2, debunking was implemented by scientists hired by the tobacco industry to create a perception of doubt regarding the risks of smoking and by HIV/AIDS researchers to identify the cause and transfer of the disease. In similar fashion, the NFL questioned Omalu's reputation and medical credentials regarding his CTE findings to attempt to discredit his research. Debunking is often used when some type of moral panic arises around a "socially perceived threat" (Vasterman, 2018, p. 20). This concern has been abundant when considering the role of media in reporting on these perceived threats (Gamson & Modigliani, 1989; Oates, 2017; Sandman, 1994; Vasterman, 2018).

Thus, the relationship between scientists and journalists has a checkered history with claims of questionable reporting of research findings, sensationalized stories, and skewed data, just to name a few overarching areas of concern often connected to public awareness (Goodell, 1987; Salleh, 2001; Sandman, 1994). This relationship is both symbiotic and dichotomous. Scientists need journalists to help move their research beyond the laboratory, and journalists need scientists to help craft news about complex topics to make stories compelling and accessible for an audience through simplified language and relevance (Brittle & Zint, 2003). However, history reveals a relationship where "interactions have often been characterized by feelings of ambivalence, mistrust, and sometimes even disdain" (Dudo, 2015, p. 762). This combative history is created through conflicting professional ideologies. This chapter offers in-depth analysis to examine how media translated science into public knowledge through its reporting of CTE.

JOURNALISTIC PURPOSE AND PROCESS

Deuze (2005) outlined five ideological tenets for journalism: public service, objectivity, autonomy, immediacy, and ethics. There is noticeable overlap between scientists and journalists regarding objectivity and ethics, given their commitment to professional integrity. However, the areas of being a public watchdog against the powerful, having autonomy to pursue topics independent of corporate or financial oversight (e.g., government or privately funded research), and the inherent need for immediacy in a news cycle are where journalistic inquiry diverges from scientific investigation. The speed and independence with which media share information is paramount to the ideology of American journalism.

These ideological functions guide a journalistic process that parallels a rhetorical approach. While Deuze provides the purpose of journalism, Shapiro (2010) describes a process guided by five journalistic faculties: (1) discovery, (2) examination, (3) interpretation, (4) style, and (5) presentation. This process begins in a linear fashion but can become cyclical based on the life cycle of a news story. Discovery is uncovering a story and deciding to pursue it. Examination is unique to journalists and is the verification of facts and testing the coherence of those facts (Kovach & Rosenstiel, 2007). Interpretation is akin to sensemaking to decipher meaning for a story. This step in the process can be challenged when navigating between a planned news story and unexpected events (Patriotta & Gruber, 2015). Style is how a journalist makes a story relevant to the reader. Finally, presentation is a collective action to create a final product that can be enhanced by where the story is placed in the newspaper and what additional elements are included (e.g., photographs, graphics, subheadings). This process positions the journalist in what Manoff and Schudson (1986) describe as a "double reality" (p. 4) where a reporter produces a story of which he or she is separate from but becomes a part of the story through the reporting process. The way a story is presented can also be influenced by cultural and ideological differences that often favor an American ideology of journalism (Barnhurst, 2014; Evans, 2016).

The process becomes clearer through repetition, but how stories emerge is rarely predictable. Through these ideological constructs, however, media play a significant role in perpetuating public events through repeated coverage of stories that gain traction in the public sphere. Molotch and Lester (1974) produced a typology of public events into four categories: (1) routine events, (2) accidents, (3) scandals, and (4) serendipity. The distinguishable characteristics between these four types of public events are how they are promoted. Routine events are the most common and are scheduled with advanced notice for media attention. Accidents are sudden and unpredictable, but if they offer long-term significance (e.g., BP oil spill, Watergate), they merge with routine events often through press briefings. Scandals can have elements of accidents and public events, which are uncovered often through dynamics of power connected with access to information and who controls it. Serendipitous events are the least common because they are unplanned public events promoted by someone, often not the perpetuator of the discovery. The type of event and what might follow can influence Deuze's purpose and Shapiro's process of journalism, especially when a story takes years to fully develop.

Any story on a newspaper's front page will be connected to one or more of these event characteristics (Molotch & Lester, 1974). That is how news media become aware of what to report (Schudson, 1989). Depending on the timeliness and unpredictable nature of a public event, journalists rely on the ideological construct of objectivity (Manoff & Schudson, 1986) to report the "material facts" (Tuchman, 1972, p. 670) provided by sources to mitigate any redress they may risk in reporting on difficult and developing stories. However, what defines material facts depend on who is reporting the story and what prior knowledge they have of any public event, which influences the way a story is framed and allows "a degree of controversy" (Gamson & Modigliani, 1989, p. 3) to emerge within a common frame.

METHODOLOGY

Since scientists identify media as a substantial driving force behind understanding and/or misconception of CTE (Carson, 2017; Kuhn et al.,

2017; Mannix, Meehan, & Pascual-Leone, 2016; Merz et al., 2017; Moon & Theodore, 2016; Perrine, Helcer, Tsiouris, Pisapia, & Stieg, 2017), the primary research in this book provides a longitudinal study of how newspapers reported about CTE. Through a mixed methods approach, how newspapers positioned CTE in its coverage provides a general understanding of the significant rise of CTE in the public domain as well as the sports, leagues, and individuals most frequently positioned alongside CTE. The mission of this research was two-fold. First, it is presented to offer a chronological snapshot of CTE's media evolution and the importance placed on CTE by media through framing concepts of selection, salience, and placement. Second, the research identified that from its infancy in the public sphere guided by journalists reporting on evolving scientific findings, CTE was framed as a scientific problem linked primarily to football with the NFL as the overriding focus.

This research examined 737 newspaper stories published between 2006 and 2017 to examine how journalists collectively positioned CTE as the science developed (or re-emerged) alongside the NFL. These stories provide an evolving look at how media reported on and framed CTE. Each news story, if examined in isolation and removed from social understanding, produces what Phillips (1976) describes as "a self-contained particle of 'reality'" (p. 89). Instead, these individual news stories provide glimpses into the mediated creation, development, and evolution of CTE. Six newspapers were included in this study: the *New York Times*, the *Washington Post*, *USA Today*, the *Pittsburgh Post-Gazette*, the San Jose *Mercury News*, and the *Denver Post*. These newspapers do not offer an exhaustive examination of newspaper reporting of CTE, but they do offer an extensive cross-section of newspapers at the forefront of reporting on CTE and a geographic dispersion that spans the United States. Additionally, a Lexis-Nexis search of U.S. newspapers that reported on CTE during the twelve years included in this study identified these newspapers as leaders in the quantity of news stories.

While this research did not focus on media bias, it is important to note that studies have positioned the *New York Times* as a "newspaper of record" that historically has been credited with leading understanding of issues of significant political and social influence (Gardetto, 1997; Gusterson, 2013). This research hoped to provide a more inclusive collection of newspapers because "the American press is not monolithic" (Zelizer, Park, & Gudelunas, 2002, p. 284). Despite criticism of the *Times* and the *Washington Post* regarding coverage of political and military topics (Bachman, 2017; Gardetto, 1997), the authors of this book felt it necessary to include the *Times* and the *Post* because of their significant place in generating public discourse. *USA Today* offered a national perspective that was not tied to one geographic location for its reporting.

It was necessary to include a Pittsburgh newspaper in this study because of the city's long-term connection to CTE from Omalu's initial finding to the movie *Concussion* as well as its position as a cultural space that exemplified an NFL city (Beissel et al., 2014). To ensure use of the most extensive reporting, the *Post-Gazette* was selected instead of the *Pittsburgh Tribune Review* despite the *Tribune Review* publishing the first—and only—identifiable story through the Lexis-Nexis search that mentioned CTE in the United States in the twenty-first century prior to 2006. After that initial report, the *Post-Gazette* published more than two and half times the amount of coverage compared to the *Tribune Review* and thus was included in this research because of that significant difference. West coast newspapers with large circulation numbers, for example the *Los Angeles Times* and the *San Francisco Chronicle,* were not accessible to the authors. Therefore, the *Mercury News* and the *Denver Post* were the most widely circulated papers in the western United States that were accessible to the authors and offered a balance of coverage in the sample to hopefully avoid any perception of east coast bias in examining how CTE was covered. Additionally, the San Jose and Denver markets offered substantial coverage of CTE because of their connection to NFL teams (San Francisco 49ers, Oakland Raiders, Denver Broncos) and several locally significant CTE storylines.

The stories for this research were identified by searching "chronic traumatic encephalopathy" through the Lexis-Nexis database. The initial search found 992 stories from the six newspapers. The first author scanned all the articles to determine relevance to include in this study, and articles were removed for multiple reasons. First, articles were excluded if they were a duplicate in the Lexis-Nexis search. Second, articles were removed if they were published multiple times by different newspapers. For example, articles originally published by the *New York Times* were recirculated by other newspapers. Additionally, syndicated columns by George Will appeared in multiple newspapers. In these instances, only the original article published in the *Times* or the first day a column by Will appeared was included. Third, if the article was a film or book review that did not include original analysis or reporting about CTE or brain injuries, then it was excluded. Fourth, only stories with a headline were included. For example, newspapers will often publish notebook sections or multiple wire stories where only the top story receives a headline. In these instances, even if CTE was in the text of a sub story, it was excluded to maintain consistent story elements for coding and further analysis. Following this search process, 75 percent of the stories identified through the initial Lexis-Nexis search were included for analysis.

DESCRIPTIVE CONTENT ANALYSIS

The authors approached the quantitative portion of this research as a descriptive content analysis. This approach was selected because this study started in the beginning of CTE reporting in mainstream media as evident by no published stories in U.S. newspapers between 1990 and 2004. Thus, to understand how media constructed CTE in its earliest phase of reporting required gathering descriptive statistics to identify trends. The advantages of this research approach were that it offered a nonobtrusive measurement of a communication process, was optimal for a longitudinal study of archival material, and reduced data to a manageable measurement technique that would be "logistically impossible for close qualitative analysis" (Riffe, Lacy, & Fico, 2005, p. 38). The findings from this quantitative coding process allowed the authors to identify a manageable number of articles to be examined more closely through qualitative analysis in chapter 6 as part of this mixed method approach.

A code book was developed by the authors to examine CTE through its mediated context. Guided by framing theory (Entman, 1993), this quantitative coding process was used to help establish how often CTE was included in stories (e.g., selection) and how prominently it was situated alongside different variables (e.g., sports leagues, other neurodegenerative diseases, side effects) to understand the context in which CTE was framed (e.g., salience). The code book included general newspaper categories: newspaper name, publication year, and the length of the article. The length of articles was important to examine if space limitations affected how CTE was framed. Short articles were defined as less than 500 words. Medium-length articles were between 500 and 999 words. Long articles were defined as 1,000 words or more.

The articles were coded for numerous variables beginning with where and how CTE and other significant categories were included in the headline and lead. The headline and lead are established journalistic signifiers intended to provide readers with the major topics discussed throughout a given text (van Dijk, 1988). This process should streamline understanding for the reader. The headline should offer "maximum out of the information flood" (Dor, 2003, p. 719), and the lead would then synthesize what was considered the most important and timely of that information. Concerns of incongruity between headline and lead or headline and text has been a concern for media researchers who have discovered a disconnect between headlines and what a story represents (Andrew, 2007; Haskins, 1966; Lagerwerf, Timmerman, & Bosschaeart, 2016; Tannenbaum, 1953). The quantitative content analysis offered an opportunity to examine for correlation between CTE and other variables throughout the reporting process.

Headlines were coded across six variables. First, the headline was coded if CTE or chronic traumatic encephalopathy appeared. Second, the headline was coded if concussion was included. Third, a category for "brain" was used, and the term was coded if brain was mentioned in conjunction with damage, disease, injury, or trauma. Fourth, a category for "head" was used, and the term was coded if head was mentioned in conjunction with injury or trauma. Disease and damage were not included in this category because these terms are used almost exclusively with long-term issues related to the brain but not the head. Lastly, headlines were coded if they included NFL (or National Football League) or NHL (or National Hockey League). While this book is focused on the NFL, with growing scientific research and media interest appearing related to hockey, it was important to code for NHL to examine how any media reporting shifted, if at all, over time.

The inverted pyramid style of news reporting was first established to assist copy editors with layout and design of the newspaper to cut off the least important information at the bottom of a story, if necessary, in the editing process. This style developed into established industry practice to summarize the most important information in the story in the first sentence and then continue telling the story in a top-down order of significance (Pöttker, 2003). Thus, the lead should offer the greatest amount of information related to the crux of the story. The lead was defined in this research as the first three paragraphs of a story to allow enough information to be included regardless of whether the story was considered a "hard news" story or a feature. The lead was coded across three variables specific to this study: CTE, NFL, or NHL. Again, these terms appear most often together in scientific literature about CTE, so it was important to examine if that translated to media coverage.

The remaining coding categories were concerned with the entire article. Multiple categories were coded to help determine how much context was provided in the stories. A category was created for "punch-drunk" and another for "dementia pugilistica" to determine if the news stories provided historical context specific to the scientific evolution of CTE. Next, eleven sports were coded to determine what sports beyond football were included in stories that mentioned CTE. These sports did not have to be discussed in direct connection to CTE. The sports included in the code book were auto racing, boxing, cheerleading, gymnastics, hockey, lacrosse, mixed-martial arts, rugby, soccer, softball, and wrestling. Auto racing included NASCAR, Indy Car, or any other mention of racing vehicles. Mixed-martial arts included MMA or UFC references.

Specific to CTE, ten side effects identified in medical literature or news stories were included in a preliminary code book. After multiple attempts for reliability, only six were included for further coding because of their clear description. These effects had to be mentioned in direct connection to CTE. The side effects included in the final code book were aggression, confusion, depression, headaches, memory loss, and suicide. Additionally, to examine how CTE was positioned in relation to other neurodegenerative diseases, the articles were coded for presence of Alzheimer's disease, amyotrophic lateral sclerosis (ALS or Lou Gehrig's disease), dementia, and Parkinson's disease. Dementia was coded only as a stand-alone disease to differentiate it from dementia pugilistica.

CODER RELIABILITY

Student coders were recruited to participate in the coding process. These students were recruited from the Zimmerman School of Advertising & Mass Communications and through the Office of Undergraduate Research at the University of South Florida. Following initial inquiry from students, seven students were accepted as part of the original cohort for coding consideration. Over the course of one month, the coders were introduced to CTE and the concepts of media framing through individual meetings to determine if they remained interested. All seven students remained and participated in two group meetings to discuss the coding process, examine multiple example articles, and practice coding the articles. Following these meetings, coders were given ten sample articles to practice coding. After two weeks, the coders met again with the lead author to discuss the coding process, raise questions about concerning topics, and collectively help to reconfigure the code book based on their interpretations and perceptions.

Following these coder training sessions, the seven coders, which included five mass communication students (three undergraduate and two graduate) and two undergraduate honors students majoring in science-related fields, were given 144 news stories for a 20 percent sample to begin coding to test for reliability. Multiple categories tested at .80 or higher, which is considered an acceptable reliability level in content analysis (Riffe et al., 2005). After the first coding session, one coder was removed from consideration due to reliability numbers too far removed from the other coders. A meeting was conducted with the six remaining coders to examine what should be included or excluded from the coding process. The coders were asked to re-code for fourteen remaining unreliable categories. During the second phase of coding, two of the remaining coders dropped out of the coding process. The four remaining coders completed the re-coding process and a few categories remained to reach reliability of .80 or higher. Six categories reached reliability of .80 or higher across three of the four coders. The other coder tested reliable above .70. These individual categories were discussed between the lead author and coders to better understand where the minor coding discrepancies occurred in the few missing articles. Following an additional meeting with the four coders to clarify any confusion related to the coding process, reliability of .80 or higher was attained for all coding categories.

Once reliability was reached for all categories, each of the four coders was given 20 percent of the remaining articles in this study. This final coding process was completed in May 2018. For their respective participation in the coding process, the coders received a research credit on their transcripts as well as a mention by name in the acknowledgement section of this book.

FREQUENCY DISTRIBUTION

These findings represent the 737 news stories published between 2006 and 2017. The *New York Times* served as the newspaper of record for CTE with more than one-third ($n = 264$, 35.8 percent) of the cumulative stories in this study, which is not surprising given the newspaper's historical track record of leading public discourse and its role in breaking the CTE story. The remaining story distribution was relatively balanced as the *Washington Post* published 110 stories (14.9 percent), *USA Today* and the *Post-Gazette* each published 109 stories (14.8 percent each), followed by the *Denver Post* ($n = 73$, 9.9 percent) and the *Mercury News* ($n = 72$, 9.8 percent). Medium length stories ($n = 330$, 44.8 percent) were the most common, followed by long stories ($n = 248$, 33.6 percent) and short stories ($n = 159$, 21.6 percent). This is a good sign that on average stories that discussed CTE provided more space to possibly include context related to a complex and developing medical condition.

Stories that mentioned CTE witnessed a precipitous rise in the aggregate number of published accounts (see figure 5.1). As previously stated, only one U.S. newspaper outside the sample of newspapers included in this study ever mentioned CTE in an article between 1994 and 2005, according to the available Lexis-Nexis database. Across the six newspapers included in this study, the evolution of CTE mentions in newspaper stories showed a steady ascension with a significant spike occurring in 2009 when the congressional hearings took place. Then another spike happened between 2011 and 2013 when several significant NFL and NHL players committed suicide and were later found to have CTE. Additionally, *League of Denial* was released in 2013 that outlined the per-

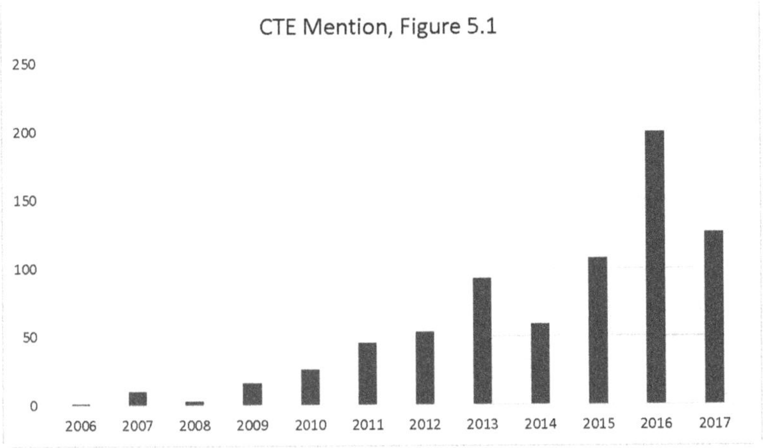

Figure 5.1. CTE mentions, 2006–2017.

ceived NFL cover-up of brain trauma. Lastly, a significant spike occurred in 2016 as CTE in the NFL reached a fever pitch amid published scientific studies on the heels of the release of *Concussion* and finally an admission by Jeff Miller of a link between CTE and football.

HEADLINE-TO-LEAD SYMMETRY

Beyond the basic mention of CTE in a story, the headline offers a unique space of analysis for three reasons. First, how often CTE was mentioned in the headline can help ascertain if a story was perceived to focus on CTE. Second, how often concussion appeared in the headline in conjunction with a story that mentioned CTE would fit into a misperception that concussions cause CTE (Carson, 2017) and thus should be linked together. Third, how often CTE and the NFL appeared in the same headline could provide a correlational link between the degenerative brain disease and football. Of the 737 stories in this study that mentioned CTE somewhere in the text, the NFL was most frequently linked via headline with nearly one-fourth (n = 170, 23.1 percent) of the headlines including the league by name or acronym (see figure 5.2). Concussion ranked second in total headline mentions (n = 144, 19.5 percent) in stories that include CTE somewhere in the text. CTE appeared in just 12.1 percent (n = 89) of the headlines associated with those stories. The brain category garnered 80 headlines (10.9 percent), followed by head and NHL, which were each mentioned in 26 headlines (3.5 percent).

More than one-third of the 144 stories that featured concussion in the headline also included a cross-reference to the NFL (n = 51, 35.4 percent).

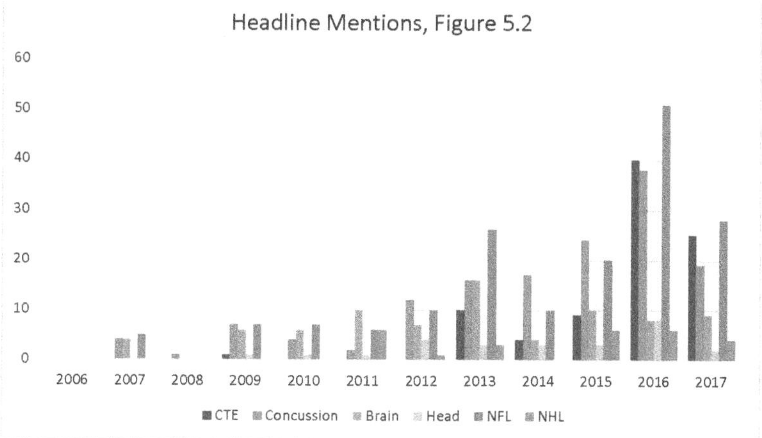

Figure 5.2. Headline mentions, 2006–2017.

Of the 89 headlines that identified CTE, only three added a cross-reference to concussion, while 27 (30.3 percent) included a reference to the NFL. Nearly one-fourth (n = 18, 22.5 percent) of the 80 stories with "brain" in the headline included a cross-reference to the NFL. Five stories overlapped brain, concussion, and CTE in headlines across these three brain-related concerns. Therefore, when all references to the three brain-related issues are accounted for collectively, more than half (n = 91, 53.5 percent) of the 170 stories that had NFL in the headline associated the league with some type of brain disease or trauma. That number only accounts for direct mentions of the league by name. The next chapter outlines how the headlines function to more implicitly link CTE specifically to football, and by large extension, the NFL.

These numbers represent two interesting findings. First, the NFL is overwhelmingly linked by media through headlines to some type of brain-related issue. Second, these newspapers collectively struggled over time with how to consistently link the league to brain injury or disease. When examining how the story written by the journalist was summarized by the editors in the headlines, the focus is somewhat split between concussion and CTE. Since concussion is the medical term more widely accepted and discussed as a sport-related brain injury, there is evidence that editors chose this more commonly understood term for public discussion. However, this could create confusion for the reader between how the headline might portray the story's focus and how the story informed the reader, especially in this sample of stories that discussed CTE in the text. Thus, the question became did the story effectively transition from headline to lead to provide an accurate summary of the text (van Dijk, 1988).

Of the stories in this study, 292 (39.6 percent) positioned CTE in the first three paragraphs. In comparison, the NFL was written in the lead in more than half of the stories (n = 394, 53.5 percent). When comparing for cross-references, the NFL was mentioned in nearly two-thirds (n = 184, 63 percent) of the 292 stories that included CTE in the lead. A Pearson-product moment correlation was used to test the relationship between CTE and the NFL in the lead. The relationship was statistically significant ($p < .01$) and positively correlated with a small strength of association (.115). This means that stories that included CTE in the lead were more likely than not to include NFL in the lead and that journalists, when reporting on CTE in the lead, connected the disease with the NFL. Considering that scientists continue to identify a wide range of other sport-related and non-sport related cases of CTE, these findings indicate a journalistic process that highlighted a distinct relationship between CTE and the NFL.

These findings explain how journalists connected CTE and the NFL in the lead, but how did the newspapers transition from headline to lead when prioritizing CTE or NFL in the headline? Of the 89 articles that included CTE in the headline, 76 of those stories (85.3 percent) included CTE in the lead and 48 (53.9 percent) positioned the NFL in the lead, which was nearly identical to the frequencies in the overall sample. A Pearson-product moment correlation was used to test the relationship between CTE in the headline against CTE and NFL in the lead. The relationship between CTE in the headline and CTE in the lead was statistically significant ($p < .01$) and positively correlated with a medium strength of association (.347). The relationship between CTE in the headline and NFL in the lead was not statistically significant and produced only a minuscule association (.004).

In the headline, NFL was the most frequently used of the coded variables. Of the 170 stories that mentioned NFL in the headline, 146 of those stories (85.9 percent) included NFL in the lead and 73 positioned CTE in the lead (42.9 percent). These findings were comparable to the translation from headline to lead for CTE as the primary variable but provided less of a relationship between the disease and the NFL. A Pearson-product moment correlation was used to test the relationship between NFL in the headline against NFL and CTE in the lead. The relationship between NFL in the headline and NFL in the lead was statistically significant ($p < .01$) and positively correlated with a medium strength of association (.356). The relationship between NFL in the headline and CTE in the lead was not statistically significant and did not reach the minimum for a small strength of association (.037).

If there is public confusion that links concussions with CTE, either via the *Concussion* movie or the often-referred to "concussion" lawsuit against the NFL, this research wanted to examine if journalists played a part in constructing that confusion. When comparing the use of concussion in the headline in 144 news stories, only three stories included CTE in the same headline, but nearly one-third ($n = 46$, 31.9 percent) included CTE in the story's lead. Since so few mentioned both in the same headline, there was no need to test for correlation. However, to test the relationship between concussion in the headline and CTE in the lead, a Pearson-product moment correlation test was used. The relationship between concussion in the headline and CTE in the lead was statistically significant ($p < .05$) and negatively correlated with minimal association (-.077). This means that headlines that included concussion were less likely to include CTE in the headline. When comparing concussion with the NFL, fifty-one positioned concussion and NFL in the same headline (35.4 percent) and nearly two-thirds ($n = 95$, 66 percent) of the stories with concussion in the headline included NFL in the lead. To test the relationship between concussion and NFL in headlines, a Pearson-product moment correlation test was used. The relationship between concussion and NFL in the headline was statistically significant ($p < .01$) and positively correlated with a small strength of association (.144). The relationship between concussion in the headline and NFL in the lead was statistically significant ($p < .01$) and positively correlated with a small strength of association (.124).

These findings indicated a successful journalistic process for creating a relationship between headline and lead where the headline achieved what Andrew (2007) called a "dual objective" (p. 28) that attracted attention through headline usage and provided a relatively accurate summary connected to the lead. The positive correlation from NFL in the headline to NFL in the lead as well as CTE in the headline to CTE in the lead provides a statistical glimpse into how newspaper editors summarized a story that journalists prepared for the reader. The negative correlation between concussion and CTE is a positive indication overall that newspapers may have reduced some level of confusion by not completely misrepresenting a connection between concussion and CTE. However, the fact that nearly one-third of the stories still created a perceived relationship does not vindicate journalists from needing to more accurately articulate how a story will transition from headline to lead.

The findings also indicated that news stories in this study produced a journalistically constructed relationship between brain trauma and the NFL through the headline and lead writing. The small correlation relationships could indicate that journalists provided additional context when positioning stories about concussions or CTE. However, these findings showed they were more likely than not to create an association between the NFL and one of these publicly (and scientifically) understood terms related to brain injuries.

PROVIDING CONTEXT

Scientific publications about CTE often (but certainly not always as previously discussed) included historical context of the disease's evolution from "punch-drunk" to "dementia pugilistica" to CTE so readers were reminded that this disease was not just concocted by Bennet Omalu but that it shifted over time to become more scientifically positioned as a degenerative brain disease that was not isolated to boxers (Cantu & Register-Mihalik, 2011). Levin and Bhardwaj (2014) explained that CTE became a more commonly referred to "nomenclature for this disease" (p. 335). Therefore, this study wanted to examine what historical context, if any, that journalists provided for CTE. Sadly, few did, as twenty-one stories (2.8 percent) mentioned punch-drunk somewhere in the story, while twelve stories (1.6 percent) identified dementia pugilistica in the story. Only four stories provided significant context by mentioning both terms. One might contend that this was a by-product of the dwindling space afforded for newspapers to print stories, but it also served as an indictment of an inability or unwillingness by journalists to provide historical context to readers.

Just as the terminology shifted from punch-drunk to CTE to be more inclusive of other sports, this study coded for other sports to provide a snapshot of which ones were included in stories that at some point referenced CTE in the text. Since some scientists pushed the notion that CTE and brain injuries were not just a football problem, this research felt it was important to see if journalists connected other sports in a similar manner. While the sport did not have to be directly linked to CTE, one can presume that many stories discussed various types of brain injuries, and thus, indirectly and discursively brought these other sports into the conversation. Hockey (*n* = 124, 16.8 percent), soccer (*n* = 91, 12.3 percent), and boxing (*n* = 65, 8.8 percent) represented the most frequently identified sports included in the stories. Lacrosse (*n* = 32, 4.3 percent), rugby (*n* = 31, 4.2 percent), auto racing (*n* = 27, 3.7 percent), and wresting (*n* = 22, 3 percent) were the only other sports that reached at least three percent of all stories in this sample. Mixed-martial arts (*n* = 18, 2.4 percent), cheerleading (*n* = 11, 1.5 percent), softball (*n* = 3), and gymnastics (*n* = 1) each were included. What was notable from these findings was an emphasis on global sports with significant professional (mostly male) presence. Hockey and soccer offer male and female versions of their respective sport. However, it can be argued that media exposure for women's hockey and soccer are primarily secluded to the Olympics and World Cup (Bell & Coche, 2018; Billings et al., 2014; MacArthur et al., 2016), and thus, would not be referenced as frequently as their male professional counterpart. With that in mind, these findings cannot be parsed out regarding possible gender difference in how those sports were positioned in the reporting, but there was a noticeable drop-off in number of references to perceived female-only sports, which was troubling.

Two other topics related to brain injuries were coded in these news stories. First, the symptoms and side effects often linked to CTE in scientific research, which have been problematized (Iverson et al., 2018), and media stories were tested for frequency and association. Second, other neurodegenerative diseases were tested for frequency and association. These topics afforded a possible opportunity for journalists to offer context alongside—and differentiation from—CTE. Symptoms and side effects were coded in direct correlation to CTE.

The other neurodegenerative diseases were coded only for presence in the story to assess how often they were brought into the reporting as more publicly and historically recognized diseases.

Suicide (*n* = 184, 25 percent) was the most frequently mentioned side effect or symptom connected to CTE. Depression (*n* = 173, 23.5 percent) and memory loss (*n* = 131, 17.8 percent) followed as most often associated with CTE. Headaches (*n* = 57, 7.8 percent), aggression (*n* = 39, 5.3 percent), and confusion (*n* = 34, 4.6 percent) were included in some reporting but did not amount to a substantial part of the conversation. Pearson-product moment correlation tests were conducted to identify how likely these side effects or symptoms were to appear with each other. The relationships between all six effects were positive with varying strengths of association, which indicated that each symptom was more likely than not to appear in association with one of the others (See table 5.1).

Each of these symptoms or side effects was coded in relation to CTE within the story's text. Of the eighty-nine stories that used CTE in a headline, suicide ($n = 32$, 36 percent), memory loss ($n = 28$, 31.5 percent), and depression ($n = 27$, 30.3 percent) were the most frequently identified symptom in those stories. Aggression followed with eleven mentions (12.4 percent) while confusion and headaches each appeared in six stories (6.7 percent). To test relationships between CTE in headlines and these symptoms, a Pearson-product moment correlation test was used. A relationship was found to be statistically significant with aggression ($p < .01$), memory loss ($p < .01$), and suicide ($p < .05$).

Of the 292 stories that referenced CTE in a lead, depression appeared most often ($n = 90$, 30.8 percent) in those stories. Suicide ($n = 84$, 28.8 percent) was next, followed by memory loss ($n = 72$, 24.7 percent). Headaches ($n = 26$, 8.9 percent), aggression ($n = 25$, 8.6 percent), and confusion ($n = 20$, 6.8 percent) each appeared in less than 10 percent of stories where CTE was in the lead. To test relationships between CTE in the lead and these symptoms, a Pearson-product moment correlation test was used. A relationship was found to be statistically significant with aggression ($p < .01$), confusion ($p < .05$), depression ($p < .01$), and memory loss ($p < .01$). The strength of association for each was small but positively correlated.

Table 5.1. Correlations

		Aggression	Confusion	Depression	Memory Loss	Headaches	Suicide
Aggression	Pearson Correlation	1	.410**	.255**	.318**	.113**	.172**
	Sig. (2-tailed)		0.000	0.000	0.000	0.002	0.000
	N	737	737	737	737	737	737
Confusion	Pearson Correlation	.410**	1	.183**	.304**	.154**	0.067
	Sig. (2-tailed)	0.000		0.000	0.000	0.000	0.067
	N	737	737	737	737	737	737
Depression	Pearson Correlation	.255**	.183**	1	.471**	.259**	.294**
	Sig. (2-tailed)	0.000	0.000		0.000	0.000	0.000
	N	737	737	737	737	737	737

Memory Loss	Pearson Correlation	.318**	.304**	.471**	1	.078*	.207**
	Sig. (2-tailed)	0.000	0.000	0.000		0.034	0.000
	N	737	737	737	737	737	737
Headaches	Pearson Correlation	.113**	.154**	.259**	.078*	1	0.056
	Sig. (2-tailed)	0.002	0.000	0.000	0.0034		0.129
	N	737	737	737	737	737	737
Suicide	Pearson Correlation	.172**	0.067	.294**	.207**	0.056	1
	Sig. (2-tailed)	0.000	0.067	0.000	0.000	0.129	
	N	737	737	737	737	737	737

Note: **=Correlation is significant at the 0.01 level (2-tailed); *=Correlation is significant at the 0.05 level (2-tailed).

Tests were conducted to examine relationships between stories and headlines that mentioned the NFL or concussions with any of the symptoms. No relationships were found to be statistically significant except for headaches with headlines, and that relationship was negatively correlated. Therefore, the symptoms associated directly with CTE were theoretically positioned in a way that was accurately reported. However, these findings indicated a possible desire to sensationalize a story when CTE was used in the headline since those stories were more likely to appear in relation to aggression or suicide, which can be perceived as the emotional, behavioral, and violent effects. Conversely, when CTE was positioned in the lead, which required a reader to look beyond the headline, the symptoms more likely to appear in association with CTE were the long-term, and perceived less violent, cognitive effects (e.g., confusion, memory loss).

Lastly, how other neurodegenerative diseases were discussed in relation to concussions, CTE, and the NFL was examined. Dementia appeared in one-third ($n = 245$, 33.2 percent) of all 737 news stories. Alzheimer's disease was discussed in nearly one-fifth ($n = 146$, 19.8 percent) of all stories, followed by ALS ($n = 62$, 8.4 percent) and Parkinson's ($n = 54$, 7.3 percent). All four of these diseases were positively correlated and statistically significant ($p < .01$). Interestingly, none of the diseases tested as statistically significant in relation to CTE and had a mix of positive and negative correlations. However, when compared to the NFL mentions in headlines, all four diseases were statistically significant and positively correlated. Regarding NFL in the lead, all four diseases were positively correlated, but Alzheimer's disease was the one that did not test as statistically significant.

FINDING THE CTE STORY

CTE and media fit neatly together over time into all four categories of the public event typology that positioned it as a socially important gap, both in scientific literature review and as a public health issue related to brain trauma (Rabinovici, 2017). Sadly, CTE has become a routine event through the sheer quantity of reported cases presented by media that were often promoted through press releases and scheduled news conferences to report the findings. However, Wheelwright (2016) cautioned against the speed with which CTE research was published, and subsequently reported on, because "feelings of urgency can prompt mistakes" (p. 20) in findings or how they were publicly represented. Despite this noted concern, CTE became a consistent news event where its origin and development in the media happened more through serendipity and accident that fueled a scandal. The scandal reached a fever pitch when the NFL was connected to CTE and brain injuries and the long-term story centered on conflict between science and football that played out through media. As Salleh (2001) noted, "journalists prefer to frame stories as conflicts between two extreme opposing viewpoints. For this reason, controversial science is very newsworthy" (p. 29). Examples of conflicts that garnered headlines and storytelling included skewed scientific findings that resulted in lawsuits, challenges of public perception, and ultimately, an admission of guilt, or at least an admission of a link between football and CTE, followed by claims that more scientific data was needed to better define that link. Conflict fueled many of the stories but a need for public understanding guided the mediating process of CTE.

The findings from the descriptive content analysis offered a glimpse into how newspapers across the United States positioned CTE in its reporting from the disease's public infancy to its rapid ascension when it reached a peak of story saturation in 2016. The increased positioning of CTE in relation to the NFL, especially in the lead, pointed to what Hippocrates (1999) described as a function of the journalistic process that "demands that one issue is prioritized over another to fit into a news story format like the inverted pyramid" (p. 65) that focuses an issue around conflict with perceived news value interpreted by editors as what the readers want.

As this quantitative analysis outlines, CTE (and other brain-related issues) was positioned in a linear relationship with the NFL. Additionally, the NFL was most often linked to side effects and symptoms associated with CTE and long-term cognitive effects. However, what this quantitative data did not distinguish was how CTE was described and framed in the writing and how it was further positioned specifically in conjunction with the NFL and, more tangentially, football. Therefore, the next chapter explores this question in greater detail through a close reading of the 89 stories that positioned CTE in the headline. This will help understand what common threads journalists used to tell the story of CTE from discovery through conflict to resolution in the way of NFL acknowledgement (Bell, 1991; Tuchman, 1976).

SIX

Beyond the Headlines

CTE and the NFL

Robert Cantu is a well-respected medical professional who has studied brain injuries in sport for decades. He is a professor of neurology and neurosurgery as well as co-founder of the CTE Center at Boston University and is the medical director for the National Center for Catastrophic Sports Injury Research at the University of North Carolina at Chapel Hill. As previously discussed, he is credited with implementing the first return-to-play guidelines regarding concussion in sport (Cantu, 1986). He holds multiple other appointments and is a consultant with the NFL as well as an advisor to the league's Head, Neck, and Spine Committee.

Cantu has been cited for being critical of the league for how it has historically handled head injuries, especially during the fourteen-part, NFL-led series in *Neurosurgery* when he was the editor for the journal's sports medicine section (Schwarz et al., 2016). For example, Cantu questioned the validity of Pellman et al.'s (2004) findings that NFL players had similar symptoms between a first and repeat concussion. Cantu raised the concern because as the authors noted in the limitations no concussion history was used, which "can be argued that this makes all comparisons suspect" (Cantu, 2004, p. 874). Cantu did publish mild support for the initial study produced by the MTBI Committee (Pellman et al., 2003) but later outlined in *League of Denial* how the journal's editor, Michael Apuzzo, published the report despite objections from Cantu and other peer reviewers (Kirk & Wiser, 2013).

His co-authored book, *Concussion and Our Kids*, provided an impetus for this book with a well-crafted statement regarding the perception and confusion between concussions and CTE.

> No head trauma is good head trauma. Yet the avalanche of publicity about concussions in recent years has distorted the connection—the public's perception of the connection—between concussions and CTE. As we understand it, CTE is caused by total brain trauma, which includes concussions but is not limited to them. (Cantu & Hyman, 2012, p. 101)

This statement summarizes two prominent ideas that help understand and discuss the findings in this chapter. First, the concept of head trauma (regardless of type, depth, location, or longevity) is not good. However, public perception, especially in a sporting context, has minimized effect or impact of the word trauma, despite its frequent use and placement in conjunction with the head or brain. Trauma has become somewhat trivialized through its vague understanding outside the medical community. Its linguistic use, especially by media, has minimized trauma, which is physical damage to arguably the body's most valuable organ—the one that has no replacement. The brain is so complex that more than fifty scientific journals include brain in their respective titles. Therefore, an argument can be made for why and how something so complex cannot be afforded the necessary space in newspaper stories and other media reports to provide proper context.

The second poignant idea from Cantu's quote gets to the primary motivation behind this book. How was a link between concussions and CTE publicly presented (or distorted) by media? What role has media played in creating any confusion? Additionally, if there was confusion, how has media attempted to distinguish CTE from concussions to help readers understand the differences? As outlined in previous chapters, scientifically there is a link between concussions and CTE, but concussions alone are not the cause and culprit of CTE. It can be a variety of effects, including multiple concussions, but there are several different brain injuries that can occur through sport, ranging from the old-school "dings" to the popularized "subconcussive blows," which have been described—and challenged—as asymptomatic, repetitive internal injuries to the brain (Asken, Sullan, DeKosky, Jaffee, & Bauer, 2017; Hazrati et al., 2013).

The confusion has been linguistic. Sharp and Jenkins (2015) recommended retiring both concussion and subconcussive from medical literature as well as from future criteria in diagnosing and discussing mild traumatic brain injuries, which could offer a more unified classification to understand the severity of an individual's brain trauma. This could help rectify the first concern that trauma has become desensitized. Regardless of how a brain injury is categorized or classified or until the terms are retired, they work together to accumulate as a cause for CTE through the scientifically stated "repeated blows to the head." For media, that is not sexy enough to report as a scientific conflict to engage with readers and move the needle. Instead, concussion, brain damage, and suicide are the terms more often portrayed by media for public understanding. Therefore, editors and journalists use them, even if it skews what are presented as the causes of CTE.

In this chapter, the eighty-nine stories that included CTE in the headline were closely examined by two authors. As the quantitative data identified, the transition from headline-to-lead-to-text can mispresent key details provided in the story. While all 737 stories included in the previous analysis are important and offer a statistical glimpse into how media positioned CTE in relation to the NFL, a deeper qualitative analysis helps examine how media framed CTE. How did media define the science and the cause of CTE? Did the stories produce a link to CTE, either through sport (e.g., football, contact sports) or science (e.g., concussions, mTBI, trauma, blows to the head)? Did they frame the disease as a football, mostly NFL, problem? Overall, what context did the stories provide about CTE that made it significant enough to be placed in the headline? Before providing the qualitative analysis, it is necessary to understand the historical function of a headline and its relationship to a story.

HEADLINE AUTHORITY

The cultural influence and power afforded to newspaper headlines cannot be understated in the journalistic process. Headlines became a mainstay for newspapers in the late 1880s (Pöttker, 2003) and served a rhetorical purpose to linguistically connect editors and journalists to readers through a short summary of what a reader should expect to learn in any given text (Bell, 1991; Lagerwerf et al., 2016). Thus, headlines served as a first facilitator in how news was consumed (Birkner, 2016). That mission has not always completed the process of accurately transferring information. Contrary to that purpose, readers wanted headlines that were relevant to them and drew their attention, not necessarily that informed them (Ifantidou, 2009). Editors were not always provided with a guide to headline writing. Instead, that skill was situated as an intuitive process that developed over a career. As Dor (2003) explained, "professional knowledge is practical, not theoretical" (p. 707). This short statement provided some clarity regarding how scientific information—that was often highly theoretical—was translated into journalistic style intended to reach a broad audience.

The placement of information in prominent locations (e.g., headlines, leads) signifies a level of importance for the reader that functions to manipulate the information provided to affect the understanding of an event that "may emphasize or deemphasize the causes or consequences of events or the properties of news actors" (van Dijk, 1995, p. 15). This emphasis begins with the headline in a streamlined process of what is perceived as the most important information first to situate the news value of a story and followed by subsequently less significant or less timely information. If historical context is provided it is likely positioned toward the end of the story. This is, in short, the inverted pyramid where a "headline sets the stage" for how a reader should enter a "frame of reference" to read the story (Tannenbaum, 1953, p. 197). Despite a push for more narrative storytelling, which is growing in popularity for traditional media, the inverted pyramid is still positioned as the dominant news structure (Johnston & Graham, 2012) with the headline as the guiding force.

In connecting headlines and head injuries, Reider (2013) referenced the newspaper headline as a method to capture reader attention that is "short and pithy, communicating a simple message" (p. 2741) related to a scientific topic such as concussions that would be better understood or examined through a slow, complex discovery process. Media does not operate within a slow pace and rarely has time to fully dissect complex issues. Stylistically, headlines are the only part of a newspaper written in the present tense to offer some level of immediacy to a story. However, the past tense writing style in a full-length text rarely allows a story to gain traction beyond the immediate and timely event that caused a story to happen. As Schudson (1986) explained, "the 'developing' story that unfolds over time offers a newspaper version of the 'continuous present' tense" (p. 89). Science often provides that slow developing story for media. CTE offers a case study that moved methodically through and across various newspapers as journalists developed "common threads" (Bell, 1991, p. 149) to construct a mediated narrative for CTE.

CTE IN THE HEADLINES

The placement of CTE in the headline "provides a lens through which the remainder of the story or article is perceived" (Tannenbaum, 1953, p. 197). These "cognitive shortcuts" (Andrew, 2007, p. 28) are the focus of this chapter to more closely examine if the shortcut reference to CTE in the headline resulted in a lengthy explanation in the story for a newly constructed brain disease. Since only one article before 2013 in the total sample included CTE in a headline, it is presumed that it was not until CTE started to gain traction in public understanding through frequent media usage that it had enough merit as an attention-grabbing element in the headlines. In relation to framing theory, as CTE was included with rapidly increasing frequency in stories from 2009 to 2012, editors placed increasing value on its reach to generate readership. In 2013, ten news stories (11.2 percent) in this sample included CTE in the headline. Following a dip in references witnessed in 2014 (n = 4) and 2015 (n = 9), CTE exploded into the headlines in 2016 with forty references, which accounted for nearly half (44.9 percent) of the headlines. In 2017, the number of headline references to CTE dropped to twenty-five.

The distribution of CTE in headlines was balanced across the newspapers included in the sample for this study. In line with its position as the newspaper of record, the *New York Times* produced the largest number of CTE references (n = 21) in headlines. The *Washington Post* published eighteen headlines that referred to CTE. The *Mercury News* provided fourteen headlines, followed by *USA Today* with thirteen, the *Pittsburgh Post-Gazette* with twelve, and the *Denver Post* with eleven.

EXPLORING THE HEADLINES

This analysis focused on four main criteria to examine from headline to text. The first area of examination was the headline. Since it was already evident that CTE was present, this research wanted to explore how CTE was framed in the headline, specifically in relation to the NFL. While the quantitative data identified that twenty-seven of the eighty-nine stories cross-referenced the NFL by name, what this chapter looked for was additional tangential, yet specific, links to the NFL and, more broadly, to football. While reading the headlines, the authors counted additional references for use of the general term "football" or for a football-specific reference, such as "hall of fame," which is the pinnacle of individual achievement in professional football. Stories were also counted if they referenced a player (current or former) by name (e.g., Frank Gifford, Junior Seau, Mike Webster) because names are used in headlines when it is presumed that a reader would recognize the name and be drawn to read the article because of that association. Lastly, if a story referenced Pop Warner, which is uniquely positioned with football in youth sport, it was included in this analysis.

The second area of examination wanted to understand who journalists most often associated with CTE. Scientifically, CTE has been linked to varying contact sports—with boxing and football receiving the significant amount of literature—military members exposed to bomb blasts, and victims of domestic violence, who have been rarely diagnosed but are considered at-risk. How often did journalists link these different groups with CTE? References were divided into two groups: football and other (which included all other contact sports, military, and domestic violence victims). Specific to football, that category was divided into whether the article suggested that CTE was *directly linked* to exposure to playing football or if the article *suggested that playing football could be related* to CTE.

The third area of examination related to a cause of CTE. Since the scientific research primarily identifies the cause of CTE as "repeated blows to the head," this research wanted to examine if journalists provided a specific cause for CTE or just inferential links to the disease. To be included as a reference to cause, the article had to explicitly identify a cause for CTE. However, it did not have to provide the scientifically accepted cause, just that it offered a cause for CTE. This category was of interest because as CTE evolved in media, how willing were journalists to accept partial science as fact in their reporting?

While repeated blows to the head are identified as a scientific cause, various types of brain injuries are often discussed in connection to football and other contact sports. Thus, an additional area of examination related to cause was more interested if the newspaper stories *suggested a link* between CTE and the varying forms of brain trauma often associated with CTE. Five questions guided this area of examination for the eighty-nine stories. The first questions asked, "Does the story suggest a link between *concussions* and CTE?" The next question was, "Does the story suggest a link between *traumatic brain injury (TBI)* and CTE?" The language between the first two questions was significant because medically, concussions and mild traumatic brain injuries are defined as the same injury and just associated with different publics: concussion with sport, TBI with military and civilians (Silverberg, Lange, & Iverson, 2016). Third, "Does the story suggest a link between *sub-concussion hits or symptoms* and CTE?" Fourth, "Does the story suggest a link between *head trauma or brain trauma* and CTE?" The use of trauma was significant for this question and could be used in conjunction with either the head or brain. The final question was, "Does the story suggest a link between *repeated blows to the head* and CTE?" For this question, multiple terms represented a form of repetition in conjunction with head hits. For example, "repeated" could also be "repetitive" or use terms that indicated *plural* acts such as "chronic," "hits," "blows," "accumulation," or "cumulative" that suggested more than one. These terms offered varying linguistic approaches for journalists to describe the same occurrence in multiple ways. This section was significant to understand if journalists offered repeated act as the most commonly accepted scientific link to what can lead to CTE.

The final area of examination wanted to understand if these news stories presented a pathological differentiation for CTE from other neurodegenerative diseases. The medical literature suggested tauopathy for CTE was unique compared to Alzheimer's, ALS, dementia, and Parkinson's based on how it disassociated from the brain caused by repeated trauma as well as where it appeared in the brain. Advances in the medical understanding allowed scientists to distinguish four stages of tauopathy for greater understanding of the advancement and severity of the disease (McKee et al., 2013). However, other scientists raised concern whether a distinct tauopathy exists for CTE caused by lack of control groups or longitudinal studies (Iverson et al., 2018; Perrine et al., 2017; Solomon, 2018). Despite the medical debate, this research wanted to examine if tau differentiation was included by journalists to provide context to readers about specific traits of CTE, as they were scientifically presented over the twelve years included in this study.

The first two authors held two separate meetings that totaled eight hours to read through the eighty-nine articles together to qualitatively analyze how CTE was framed in these stories within the context outlined across the four areas of examination. The articles were read together to answer the framing questions. Additionally, this research approach allowed space and time to discuss any possible discrepancies with how to interpret the articles and how they linguistically situated CTE. The findings are divided into the four areas of examination for discussion and are primarily intended to better understand how CTE was framed in U.S. newspapers. The NFL, because of its historically and scientifically constructed relationship with CTE, became a by-product of this framing analysis as suggested from the findings in chapter 5.

FINDINGS

Headlines as Persistent Pattern

To understand the scope and magnitude of how often CTE is related to the NFL and football, a close reading of the eighty-nine headlines indicated that sixty of those stories (67.4 percent) had an explicit reference to football, with fifty-five of those connected to the NFL, which was more than double the number of references identified in the quantitative analysis. Of the twenty-eight additional headlines that connected CTE with the NFL, the references primarily included mention of individual players, who were newsworthy enough to be recognized by their name alone. These players fit into one of three categories: (1) well-known retired star (e.g., Frank Gifford, Ken Stabler); (2) a player who was connected to a headline-grabbing murder (e.g., Jovan Belcher, Aaron Hernandez); or (3) a living player who claimed to be diagnosed with CTE or indicated that they were destined for a diagnosis (e.g., Tony Dorsett, Ronnie Lott). Five headlines connected CTE directly to football, not specifically the NFL. Three of the five identified football by name and the other two referenced a lawsuit settled by Pop Warner.

Regarding the remaining twenty-nine stories that did not include football references, thirteen of those stories positioned CTE alongside another contact sport either through a specific reference to a league or athlete, which further served to construct CTE as a sport-specific disease. The NHL (three) and BMX (two) were the only other sports included in multiple headlines connected to CTE. Thus, the headlines framed CTE as only linked to contact sport both through inclusion of sporting references and the complete exclusion of either military or domestic violence victims (Gitlin, 1980; Entman, 1993).

These findings overwhelming identified a strong association between CTE and the NFL generated by newspaper headlines that created "heightened scrutiny of the practice of collision sports, particularly American football" (Mannix et al., 2016, p. 486). By frequently positioning CTE in headlines connected to football, media further perpetuated a publicly connected link between the sport and the disease. Newspapers, through the headlines, framed CTE as a football problem witnessed by a "persistent pattern" (Gitlin, 1980, p. 7) over time through the selection and emphasis on football along with minimized recognition of other contact sports and complete exclusion of other potential links to CTE. Thus, the headlines "brought an otherwise amorphous reality into a meaningful structure" (Carter, 2013, p. 3) through repeated association.

Framing CTE as a Football Problem

Science journals have published countless articles about CTE in sport, which, by extension, has guided a mediated positioning of CTE as primarily a sports-related disease. However, several researchers have connected CTE to blast exposure for military members (Goldstein et al., 2012; McKee et al., 2013; Omalu et al., 2011) and one case related to domestic violence (Roberts, Whitwell, Acland, & Bruton, 1990). Moreover, Cantu suggested a likely connection between CTE and many victims of domestic violence (Tanner, 2016) but pointed out that brains have not been donated to confirm any such speculation. Since postmortem diagnosis has historically been the only verifiable method, most often discovered through a donated brain, it was perceived by this research that the at-risk group of domestic violence victims would need a windfall of willing families to offer their brains for examination. Nevertheless, this research wanted to identify how newspapers framed CTE and explore if these stories offered context that expanded CTE beyond the athletic arena and into civilian and military life. The succinct answer was no. Journalists did not go deeper in its reporting beyond sports.

Of the eighty-nine articles that situated CTE in the headline, nineteen of the associated stories (21.3 percent) suggested that football was to blame for long-term CTE diagnoses. What was interesting in these stories was that some did not include repeated head trauma as an intermediary between football and CTE. Rather, these stories simply framed that football was to blame for CTE. Other stories positioned concussions as an intermediary between football and CTE, which was problematic for what causes CTE. While nineteen stories offered a direct link between football and CTE, another fifty stories strongly inferred that a link existed between football and CTE but was not yet definitive. Thus, sixty-nine of the eighty-nine stories (77.5 percent) that included CTE in the headline connected football to CTE either as a related-effect or as a direct cause-and-effect.

Journalists did not shy away from direct accusations against the NFL, yet they often misrepresented an association between CTE and concussions. Jenkins (2014) produced the most damning comparison between the NFL and the coal industry that required government intervention to save its employees. She wrote, "Concussions are the black lung of the NFL. And the league knows it" (p. D1). Campbell and Walker (2016) provided another example of a direct link between football and CTE, but one that misdirected the issue to "the contentious issues of concussions" whereby the NFL "relented on a once steadfast stance" (p. 2B) by publicly admitting a direct link between football and CTE, which is discussed at length in the final chapter. This issue of repeatedly connecting concussions with CTE is discussed in the next section as problematic from a scientific approach.

In stories that related CTE with football, two primary barriers affected journalists' ability or desire to draw a direct effect. First, incomplete science was cited as a limitation to offer readers with direct causality. For example, Maese (2014) wrote, "Class attorneys who filed an initial complaint linking football with CTE told the court Wednesday (November 19, 2014) the science is too incomplete to draw definitive lines and establish causation" (p. D5), but he predicted within ten years that CTE would become a regular diagnosis in living people. Second, some stories inferred a link between football and CTE but allowed the NFL's public relations machine to challenge, or at least question, scientific findings. From a journalistic standpoint, this can be presented as objectivity by allowing the league to question possible data but raised long-standing ethical questions of allowing powerful sources to dictate coverage (Sigal, 1986; van Dijk, 1988). Creating space for possible dissension raised comparisons to when Big Tobacco was pressed about links between smoking and cancer and used a defense that smoking did not guarantee a cancer diagnosis. Regardless, the probability of smoking causing cancer was ultimately proven to be a statistically greater risk than without smoking. Despite mounting evidence of CTE, even if gathered through convenience samples, this journalistic space for dissension was problematic.

Beyond football, twenty-one stories (23.6 percent) presented other contact sports, military, or domestic violence as linked to CTE. However, many of these references were substantiated through a connection with football. One example of tangential mentions situated CTE as "the disease that has reduced dozens of former football players—and soccer players and hockey players and members of the military—to shadows of themselves" (Armour, 2016, p. 3C). Two stories provided substantial space that outlined CTE as prominent in military members. Even then, the effects were positioned in related context to sport. For example, Roth (2013) wrote, "the blast effect is equivalent to several smaller blows that athletes would get playing football, hockey or other contact sports" (p. A-1). It was not until December 15, 2015, that any story mentioned victims of domestic violence as possibly at risk for CTE, and the mention was in passing.

Causal Link

Moving beyond the headline and who was associated with CTE, this research wanted to understand if—and how—newspapers dissected the scientifically complex topic of CTE in detail. It is important to recognize this section focused on the disease and not sport. As Goodell (1987) explained, the role of media was to inform—not educate—about science, and they often limited how much background information reached the public. To better understand this journalistic process, this study explored if the news stories offered a cause for CTE. If so, what was the cause? Conversely, if a story did not offer a cause but inferred a link to a specific type of brain injury, which one was most frequently associated with CTE? These questions serve to better understand if newspapers filtered information, how did it position published, scientific understanding in its reporting? Moreover, was the information "variable and sometimes even contradictory" (Goodell, 1987, p. 586)?

Less than one in five articles (n = 14, 15.7 percent) that identified CTE in the headline offered an explicit cause of the disease. The specific use of "cause" was significant in this examination. The basic understanding of "cause" is to *make something happen*. Rhetorical authority was provided by this linguistic choice and many journalists chose to not offer that scientific detail to its readers. Within the fourteen articles, it was important to explore how the journalists attributed cause and if it aligned with scientific research. Eleven of the fourteen articles accurately reflected the scientific understanding that a repetitive act of trauma to the head was a cause that resulted in CTE. A few examples included "repeated blows to the head," "repeated brain trauma," and CTE was caused "both by big hits and a number of smaller, repetitive ones." The stories that did not match the scientific causation were close but vague. One close explanation was provided in a quote by actor Will Smith, who portrayed Bennet Omalu in the movie *Concussion*, that related cause to sport. Smith said about the movie, "it's going to change the way people see football, other sports that cause CTE." The other two stories referenced that CTE was a result of "head trauma." However, these stories failed to indicate repetition and that there was "no idea how many hits cause it" but still offered that hits to the head can result in CTE. The significant finding was that newspapers, on the occasions that they did provide a cause, were accurate in their reporting.

Beyond offering an explicit cause, media suggested several links to CTE using science terminology that defined various types of brain injuries (e.g., concussion, TBI, subconcussive, or repetitive). These findings offered significant variation in how journalists positioned a link to CTE and how it might occur. Within the eighty-nine articles that included CTE in a headline, nearly half of the stories suggested a link between either "trauma" ($n = 43$) or "concussion" ($n = 42$) and CTE. Conversely, "subconcussive" ($n = 8$) and "traumatic brain injury" ($n = 5$) were rarely linked to CTE. These findings were interesting for two reasons. First, journalists elected to use more commonly understood medical terms to avoid language that sounded too scientific, which would require further explanation to provide to readers. Second, these findings supported the assertion from Cantu and Hyman (2012) that the overwhelming use of trauma and concussion in relation to CTE further served to shift public perception of a causal link to those causes. Additionally, with such limited use of TBI, which is the more civilian definition of a brain injury, these stories further positioned CTE as a sport-related issue by focusing on concussions as a link to CTE.

These findings were problematic regarding journalistic accuracy. Since concussions can lead to potential CTE diagnosis but are not the only link to the disease, overwhelming readers with mentions of concussions created a false perception of causation. Multiple stories cited the NFL's research of a decrease in concussions, which allowed space for the league to influence the conversation toward concussions and away from CTE. Additionally, the release of the *Concussion* movie produced a spike in the number of mentions of concussion beginning in 2015 that further strengthened an association between concussions and CTE. Prior to the release of the movie, newspapers were doing an adequate job of properly situating CTE in conjunction with repeated hits to the head, not just a diagnosed concussion.

Specific to the repetitive function of brain injuries providing greater potential risk for CTE, fifty-six of the stories suggested a link between some type of repetitive hits to the head and CTE. This finding indicated that when newspapers offered details about the scientific understanding of CTE, they provided a relatively accurate depiction. However, there was little consistency in the varying ways they described the repetition and how it was linked to the head or brain. A few examples were "repeated concussions," "repeated head injuries," "repeated head trauma," "countless hits," "several smaller blows," and "thousands of head collisions." This was repeatedly a linguistic challenge among journalists for how to consistently present CTE in its proper context.

Tauopathy—what makes CTE unique?

Newspapers did an adequate job of explaining that repeated blows to the head were linked as a likely cause for CTE. However, newspapers did a minimal job of moving beyond that basic context to offer readers an explanation of how CTE was scientifically distinguished from other neurodegenerative diseases, at least as defined by the scientists who supported the advancement of CTE research and were most often cited by journalists. Those researchers offered that it was the tauopathy that made CTE unique from other diseases. First, it is important to note that every human being has tau in their brain. Therefore, it is not the presence of tau that is significant. What makes CTE unique is the pathology of tau deposits that break loose from the normal protein in the brain caused by brain trauma. Those deposits then become tangled in the brain in places where tau is not usually located and thus is presented as different from Alzheimer's, ALS, dementia, and Parkinson's. In layman's terms, the unique tauopathy describes where tau appears in a postmortem brain and what path it took to get there.

Of the eighty-nine articles closely examined, seventeen of those stories (19.1 percent) mentioned tau. Most of these stories simply stopped at a simple mention of tau or tau protein in conjunction with CTE or that it signified the presence of CTE. Minimal context was offered for what tau is, what it means scientifically, or how it differentiates CTE from a neuropathological perspective. Thus, some journalists did due diligence to include what makes CTE unique but did not distinguish why. Goodell (1987) stated that a journalist's job is not to educate by translating science but to inform. However, in the case of how to distinguish CTE from other neurodegenerative diseases, especially when other scientists questioned whether CTE was truly unique, journalists could have provided some space to provide at least a basic scientific explanation and delineation.

Yet, one article did a remarkable job in outlining that tau was not unique to CTE or to football or to sport. Instead, it was ubiquitous.

> We all have tau in our brains. Normally, it makes up part of the skeleton of our brain cells. But in Alzheimer's disease, CTE and some other conditions, the tau becomes damaged and forms tangles and clumps. There is some evidence that this toxic form of the protein can then infect nearby cells, hastening its spread through the brain.
>
> Researchers like Drs. Omalu and McKee knew that the tau they were seeing in CTE was not Alzheimer's because it was showing up in different parts of the brain and advancing with different patterns. (Roth, 2013)

These two paragraphs provided a roadmap and a clear visual image for the reader, in describing both tau and how the pathology of CTE was different from other neurodegenerative diseases caused by the unique displacement of tau. Roth deserved credit for this detailed description. However, it was disappointing that it was only in 2013 that this differentiation was offered, especially as other scientists started to challenge the accuracy or validity of tau's unique quality in CTE.

Beyond Roth's expert description, Belson (2016) outlined how a new blood test could assist in detecting the protein associated with tau as a potentially cost-effective way to screen for CTE rather than more expensive neuro-imaging tests. That is, can a test can accurately diagnose CTE in living people, which has been reported but still required postmortem confirmation after death? Belson properly raised potential ethical concerns when it identified that the technology for the blood test was created by Quanterix, which was partially funded by the NFL. Therefore, the reporting provided more detail about tau and how its progression was unique but also that full understanding of CTE was likely years in the future.

With an exception for these two examples of in-depth discovery of tau, the overall reporting merely explained tau as connected to CTE and moved on. As media framing of CTE evolved, it moved more toward explanation, denial, and admission of guilt. Over time, stories did less description of CTE, its causes, and its uniqueness. Therefore, without reading these stories as a collective historiography of the tauopathy of CTE, readers were left to understand tau as something unique to CTE only in a sporting—and primarily, football—context and that tau only appeared or developed because of repeated hits to the head caused by sport.

Overall, journalists included in this research did a commendable job of taking a complex and rapidly developing topic—at least through reporting of scientific findings with minimal historical context—and attempting to dilute it for readers to understand. However, as chapter 5 outlined, the mere presence of varying phrases and topics connected to CTE was not enough. Simply mentioning "repeated blows to the head" or "tau," for example, did not explain why these things mattered or their respective role in the emergence of CTE. Thus, a deeper qualitative examination of media framing guided by the headlines was necessary to position ways in which audiences may interpret the stories being told.

Concussions and dementia had a lengthy history with the league through lawsuits and medical funding provided to former players. Thus, long-term loss of cognitive function was not new to the NFL when the newspapers in this study began printing stories about CTE in 2006. Therefore, it was important to examine why CTE reached the headlines at a more substantial rate than, say, Alzheimer's or Parkinson's. The likely reason is that CTE was something uniquely connected to the NFL, despite, of course, the eighty-plus years of research that positioned it alongside boxing. As a media storyline, CTE offered the sexy, headline-grabbing acronym that became a cautionary tale of football.

Subsequently, newspapers framed CTE as a sports-related disease connected to repeated blows to the head, with concussion as the brain injury most often associated with it. The rhetorical function of the journalistic process allowed space for different ways of saying the same thing.

Regarding CTE's causation or pathology, the newspapers in this study utilized leeway to position CTE in language that was easier to understand but could cause confusion regarding an actual cause-and-effect relationship. Overall, this research assessed that journalists did an adequate job in how they framed CTE based on interpretation of scientific findings but still created some confusion based on the varying ways it described how CTE happened. More conclusively from headline-to-text, these eighty-nine stories framed CTE as a football problem. The next two chapters explain how media framing from newspapers affected long-term understanding of CTE. First, an analysis of three films helps understand how visual media interpreted, translated, and advanced these journalistic findings about CTE. Second, as media collectively positioned CTE as a football problem, it simultaneously challenged and reified football's masculine grasp in media through the exclusion of female athletes and other at-risk collision sports.

SEVEN

Creation and Critique of Violence

Film and Football

It has been more than a decade since CTE entered public discourse (or re-entered based on decades of published science). Media played a significant role in that re-entry process as they constructed and framed *a story* about CTE through inclusion and exclusion of information, outlining cause-and-effect and the expansion of CTE beyond the NFL, while still retaining the NFL as the core entity at stake regarding long-term effects. Daily news reporting was trapped within a constant battle of an immediate need for information versus context. Immediacy has arguably provided the greatest struggle for an industry often considered the first, not final, draft of history (Zelizer, 2008). However, examining CTE coverage from incubation to consistent reporting over time allowed a glimpse into an *evolving draft* of history that changed with every new story spawned by a published scientific study or sadly another player's death, just to name two primary examples. Through the evolution of the newspaper reporting outlined in the previous two chapters, a cultural shift in media representation of CTE identified how media often straddle between two ideological tenets: journalistic objectivity and a subjective stance to challenge the validity of a sport with the strongest link to American identity. Additionally, journalists—and influential op-ed writers—even called for parents to not allow their children to play the sport, yet they rarely questioned media's role in perpetuating the sport's longevity under a guise of mediated duty to report on the games. Thus, sport journalists specifically struggled with reporting wins and losses versus life and death.

Fortuna (2015) explained, "sports media hold tremendous power to mold people's outlooks, actions, and beliefs" (p. 83). However, "sports media" have never been one holistic group. Instead, media encompassed an industry guided across various modalities, institutions, and content. Additionally, media have become cyclical purveyors of information who also served as participants in a process of sensemaking both for themselves and public understanding. Grossberg, Wartella, Whitney, and Wise (2006) described this simultaneous act as "mediamaking" through various relationships "of reciprocal influence" (p. 7) that are constructed and perpetuated through shared information.

During the 12 years of newspaper reporting examined in this book, one emergent space of crossover mediamaking was film. Three specific films—*Head Games* (2012), *League of Denial* (2013), and *Concussion* (2015)—spawned from the scientific and mediated rise of brain injuries and CTE into public discourse. These films are situated within a reciprocal relationship with newspapers at an intersection with sport. Each film was influenced by newspaper reporting but also influenced how newspapers subsequently reported on the findings offered by these new forms of mediated discourse. All three films were based on books written by people whose voices played a significant role in the collective CTE story being told. While this could have raised some concerns regarding the vantage point (and perceived bias) of each film, they relied upon in-depth reporting of brain injuries in sport that newspapers did not have the time, space, or desire to unfold.

These accounts, while limited to three, offered a style of "slow news" that provided greater context than their newspaper counterparts. Ricketson (2016) outlined "slow news," through book-length journalistic accounts that examined media coverage of the bombing of Hiroshima during World War II and the Iraq war of the 1990s, that afforded reflective "time to begin seriously contemplating the magnitude of the event" (p. 514) both for mediamakers and viewers. In no way have the authors of this book intended to compare CTE to the global magnitude of those life-changing historical events. Instead, it was Ricketson's idea of time and space to assist in the human processing of complex and evolving news stories that was a significant takeaway. Thus, the intersections of media, sport, and the popular culture form of film became intertwined in a "slow news" space of interpretation, even though the information still developed over a relatively short span of time. Additionally, these films were influenced by economic and political partners (e.g., Congress, NFL) that were situated in historical and cultural contexts of masculinity embedded in the production of sport for public consumption (Grossberg et al., 2006). Ultimately, these three films collectively challenged these masculine ideals.

To better understand the mediated role of film in the slow news process, this chapter is outlined in three parts to examine how film historically helped construct, and in the present possibly deconstruct, the masculine ideological force of football. First, a brief review of the rise of NFL Films outlines how the league used film to construct football as a masculine, yet artistic, identity. Second, the use of film—particularly documentaries—as a mode of critique explains how the same form of media once used to highlight the NFL as visual artistry could present a range of scientific counternarratives. Third, the three films were analyzed to assess how they collectively framed CTE as a football problem.

NFL FILMS AS ART

Football drama situated neatly into film with its winners and losers, protagonists, underdogs, violence, pageantry, and cultural influence on society. The NFL as a visual property began in the 1950s through broadcast television and that relationship has generated billions of dollars in revenue for the league. However, the NFL's presentation of football as an art form started in 1964 when the league purchased Blair Motion Pictures from Ed Sabol, who first produced weekly highlight films beginning in 1962 that impressed then-commissioner Pete Rozelle with the cinematic production quality (Vogan, 2013). Sabol remained as president of NFL Films and alongside his son, Steve Sabol, elevated the visual imagery of the NFL like no other sports league has ever witnessed and "fundamentally redefined the mediated production of sport" (Butterworth, 2014, p. 208). What NFL Films also accomplished was an up-close view of the violent struggle embedded in the league's on-field combat (Oriard, 2007).

Long before NFL Films was critically analyzed for its controlled and orchestrated role in NFL identity formation, the Sabols produced *They Call It Pro Football* in 1966 as the seminal work of how football could be portrayed. This film is credited with revolutionizing how football was visually produced as a long-form narrative beyond basic highlight packages (Carter, n.d.) and influenced how media corporations like HBO and ESPN situated the sports documentary as a popular broadcast genre (Vogan, 2013). Thus, the NFL served as the first sports media corporation, despite not being perceived as one in comparison to the league's network partners, to capitalize on these storylines through the creation of NFL Films. From its formative years, NFL Films not only situated football as an American cultural icon, but it promulgated the game for its militaristic comparisons and formations that constructed heroic narratives that resonated well into the twenty-first century (Butterworth, 2014; Oriard, 2007; Vogan, 2013).

They Call It Pro Football influenced "how the NFL would be perceived around the globe" (Carter, n.d., para. 1) and helped position "pro football's unique centrality to and popularity in the 1960s American culture" (Vogan, 2014, p. 36). Butterworth (2014) described these ideological underpinnings produced by NFL Films as struggle, embodied sacrifice, and spectacle that situated the game and its combatants during war times to promote patriotism in and through sport. Just as films have historically promoted U.S. military through mythological representations, Vogan (2013) described NFL Films' "overall mission to create a positive and salable mythology for the league that insulates its parent company from the criticism it continually—and often very deservedly—faces for its violence, labor practices, and other negative attributes" (p. 287). *They Call It Pro Football* served as an artistic rendering of the aesthetic and cultural values placed on American football and was "one of the all-time great masters of illusion" (Oriard, 2007, p. 18) produced through the lens of NFL Films.

Despite these critiques of NFL Films, *They Call It Pro Football* was recognized in 2012 by the Library of Congress for inclusion in the National Film Registry. In its press release, the Library of Congress anointed the film as "a mold for subsequent productions by NFL Films and has well earned its characterization as the 'Citizen Kane' of sports movies" ("2012 National Film," 2012), citing an oft-used reference credited to Steve Sabol placing NFL films on par with Orson Wells's 1941 award-winning film (Oriard, 2007; Vogan, 2013). A *60 Minutes* story in 2004 reiterated the authority granted to NFL Films "that has turned the controlled anarchy of football into money and art" (Leung, 2004, para. 3), which reinforced Murphy's (1999) assertion that NFL Films was "perhaps the most effective propaganda organ in the history of corporate America" (p. 82). Thus, through film, the NFL offered a constructed narrative of violence that was culturally and publicly accepted for years before any other film produced a modern depiction of the sport's long-term repercussions. Ironically, the inclusion of *They Call It Pro Football* as a historical relic in 2012 coincided with the release of *Head Games*, which was the first of three films included in the forthcoming analysis.

FILM AS CRITIQUE

While NFL Films constructed a specific narrative, documentary film has offered a different perspective beyond the glorified, cinematic representation the league would prefer the public to see. Nichols (1991) described that beyond fiction, "documentary offers access to a shared, historical construct. Instead of *a* world, we are offered access to *the world*. The world is where, at the extreme, issues of life and death are always at hand. History kills" (p. 109). Bruzzi (2006) raised a significant question of whether documentaries are produced as representation or record of truth regarding authenticity. Ultimately, film has provided a "record from an alternative perspective" (p. 16) that has produced a relationship between a film, its viewers, and whatever archives, documents, and/or newsreels that provided visual context. Additionally, viewer interpretations of meaning through films vary based on when and how they view the story and within what context.

As media coverage of injuries in sport has increased and evolved with more specificity, the release of each new film could be viewed with a greater amount of knowledge surrounding the risk of injuries in sport, especially regarding brain injuries. Thus, film has helped transport viewers into a space occupied by athletes beyond the playing field and stadiums filled with fans. The films in this chapter are discussed with a shared, historical understanding of brain injuries and the long-term effects on players during and after their playing careers that has come to the public forefront and to counter the mythical narrative once visually produced during NFL Films' rise to prominence.

Films about the NFL, and football in general, have previously worked to glorify the league and sport for fighting through adversity, winning as underdogs, and highlighting teamwork. Rarely has film provided a critique of the dark side of the sport. However, one film is important to understand that exposed the NFL and outlined the power of documentary film as a space for critique and rebuttal. In January 1985, HBO televised *Disposable Heroes: The Other Side of Football* that chronicled life after football and the hardships players suffered after their playing careers. The film was described as "less an angry documentary than a candid and compassionate one, caringly and skillfully shaped into a pointed statement about the seldom-reported-on-TV downside of organized sport" (Rosenberg, 1985, para. 13). The documentary aired one week before Super Bowl XIV when the Joe Montana–led San Francisco 49ers defeated Dan Marino and the Miami Dolphins, 38–16, which was the first of San Francisco's four Super Bowl titles during their 1980s dynasty.

Disposable Heroes specifically chronicled the painful reality for two former NFL lineman that followed reaching football's pinnacle. Jim Otto was a center for the Oakland Raiders from 1960–1974 and was elected to the Pro Football Hall of Fame in 1980. He was arguably the gold standard for his position until Mike Webster finished his playing career. Roger Stillwell played three seasons in the NFL with the Chicago Bears from 1975–1977 until a knee injury cut short his career. The documentary juxtaposed their stories of dealing with a lifetime of pain. The film also included interviews with Hall of Fame players O. J. Simpson and Gene Upshaw, coach John Madden, and several other players, but the focus remained on Otto and Stillwell and explored what the film's narrator described as a "dangerous and exotic trade" learned at the high school and college level. This training resulted in brief playing careers and produced "few marketable skills (while) most will be plagued with football injuries for the rest of their lives." This film does not take the league to task but offered real images of the pain that followed the glory.

Stillwell candidly explained, "In the NFL, you're always looking over your shoulder because you're disposable, you're dispensable." Just six years after his playing career, the film documented a life of five-day-a-week physical therapy sessions, his need to constantly wear a back brace, and injuries described by his parents that "completely crippled and hobbled" their son. Kyle Stillwell, Roger's wife since college, outlined that they envisioned a lavish lifestyle perpetuated by media. Instead, the glorification of sport "didn't end up that way at all," and she is shown applying ice packs to her husband's back before he was relegated to the couch for the remainder of the day. Stillwell recounted his final NFL play as "my career is laying there in the bottom of a pile."

Stillwell suffered similar pain to Otto, despite a ten-year difference in playing careers. In one compelling scene, Otto met with an orthopedic surgeon and recounted thirteen knee surgeries between his freshman year of college and the following two decades. After rehashing his medical history, Otto said, "I've had my share. I've paid my price." The doctor asked, "Was it worth it?" Otto responded, "Well, I can't do anything today. That part of it's not worth it. I had a lot of fun. I enjoyed football. It was my game, but right today, I can't be on my feet to work or anything." Like Webster's "Iron Mike" nickname, Otto was described by Madden, his former coach, as an "ironman" and that "an ironman pays for it later."

Disposable Heroes documented these hardships and used NFL Films footage against the league, where the slow-motion replays of crushing hits offered a visual reminder of the sport's brutality over its grace. The film raised concerns of an alarming use of painkillers to keep players on the field before the game's toll caught up to twenty- and thirty-year-old bodies. Sally Otto, Jim's wife, explained that in the moment she "never even gave it a second thought" to help Jim battle through a week of painful recovery at home to maintain enough strength to play on Sundays. It perpetuated a contradiction between game film and reality. Stillwell concluded the film that "when I dream, it's the old me" until he woke up to realize he was nearly crippled from the game he still wished to play.

Bodily injuries, pain, and a lifetime of rehabilitation carried the film. Sadly, *Disposable Heroes* exemplified what King et al. (2014) explained as a lifestyle where "pain—an entirely subjective phenomenon—has become vulnerable to relentless medical objectification" (p. 262) that seems acceptable in sport, despite knowledge of long-term effects. Ironically, this significant film focused on the body and presented only one mention of head injuries. Otto recounted that he had *over thirty concussions* during his time as an offensive lineman. He provided no other information and seemed to clearly recall stories throughout the film. In its time, *Disposable Heroes* did a remarkable job of questioning the value of American football versus physical, long-term toll on the body, but it would be nearly three decades before another film would critique football and other contact sports at a deeper level than the physical brutality of the body.

As focus shifted toward reinvigorated scientific research about brain injuries in sport, the impact of damage to the brain moved public dialogue beyond the threat of football to repairable and replaceable body parts, as detailed in *Disposable Heroes*, to the body's most valuable commodity. As newspapers continued to increase their reporting of concussions in football, film followed that lead into the story of CTE driven largely by timeliness and human interest (Sandman, 1994) at an intersection of conflict (scientists vs. the NFL) that produced a "*newsworthy* and saleable story" (Salleh, 2001, p. 29). Following the deaths of several high-profile professional football players, an availability cascade formed through increased published research on concussions and CTE, recognition by living athletes about the long-term effects, and on-going discussion of contact in youth sports that fueled a public debate and generated a space for film to enter the conversation.

A short summary is offered for each film. They are organized in chronological order: *Head Games*, *League of Denial*, and *Concussion*. Following the film summaries, the analysis is thematically organized to situate where these three films aligned and diverged.

Head Games *(2012)*

Head Games was a ninety-five-minute documentary that explored head injuries in sport, ranging from football and hockey to soccer and wrestling. Inspired by Chris Nowinski's 2007 book, *Head Games: Football's Concussion Crisis from the NFL to Youth Leagues*, the documentary offered a relatively linear timeline of the issue of brain trauma in sport through Nowinski's personal experience with concussions and several leading (or at least most often quoted) medical experts in the field. The film provided a big-picture exploration of how head trauma impacts athletes at all levels but offered Nowinski, former NHL player Keith Primeau, and U.S. women's soccer player Cindy Parlow Cone as cautionary tales who struggled with being advocates for safe play embedded in a culture of former athletes who miss their sport. Journalist Alan Schwarz, who is credited with breaking the concussion crisis in mainstream media for the *New York Times*, is prominently featured in the documentary as well.

Nowinski's connection to sport and brain trauma is outlined in chapter 3. Primeau played fifteen years in the NHL until he retired in 2006 following a concussion that caused him to miss all but nine games in the 2005–2006 season. During his career, Primeau scored 266 goals and amassed 1,541 penalty minutes playing primarily with the Detroit Red Wings and the Philadelphia Flyers. According to hockeyfights.com, Primeau was involved in seventy-nine career fights. Parlow Cone was a two-time college national player of the year for the University of North Carolina at Chapel Hill, a member of the 1999 U.S. Women's World Cup championship team, and a three-time Olympic medalist from 1996–2004. She retired from competitive soccer in 2006 citing post-concussion symptoms of headache and fatigue and partnered with Nowinski's Sports Legacy Institute to challenge the use of heading in soccer (Macur, 2014).

Director Steve James was best known for *Hoop Dreams,* a 1994 documentary that followed two Chicago high school basketball players that examined race and inner-city youth sports. Malec (1995) described *Hoop Dreams* as "a powerful commentary on the sports-school connection in American society" (p. 309) that perpetuated a myth beginning in youth sport that emphasized potential to reach a professional career in sport. Malec described this as more illusion than dream based on the minute statistical percentage of achieving a professional player career. However, the film's mainstream media acclaim was not echoed in academic literature that questioned the film's authenticity (Arthur & Cutler, 1995), its moral compass (Robbins, 1997), and racial disparities between white filmmakers and black teenagers (Davis, 1999). Where *Hoop Dreams* succeeded was in reaching a pinnacle as the highest-grossing documentary film for 16 years ("Top-US-grossing," 2015). It also interjected youth sport into more mainstream conversations about exposing children to trappings of the illusionary dream. *Head Games* followed a similar approach of dream versus reality.

Friedman (2016) offered that *Head Games* has potential but gets bogged down in a battle for who can be the CTE expert among leading medical professionals. Friedman was critical that this film failed if its goal was to assist in "taking down big boys like the NFL and NHL" (p. 99). While the film had its storytelling flaws, it provided a starting point for when and how CTE entered popular culture through film. Thus, it was important to include *Head Games* in any discussion of how CTE was portrayed beyond traditional mainstream media because it offered a glimpse into what individuals like Nowinski, Cantu, and McKee were doing at the forefront of this NFL crisis.

League of Denial *(2013)*

League of Denial: The NFL's Concussion Crisis (2013) was a one-hour, fifty-three-minute documentary that exposed the NFL for its consistent and repeated attempts to deny a link between football and long-term cognitive issues for players. It can be argued NFL players were—and will likely remain—an especially at-risk demographic for repeated blows to the head sustained well beyond a "normal" playing career that ends for more than 93 percent of high school football players who do not compete at the college level or beyond ("Estimated probability," n.d.). The film first appeared on the *PBS* "Frontline" series in conjunction with the release of the book by a similar title, *League of Denial: The NFL, Concussions, and the Battle for Truth,* written by ESPN investigative reporters and brothers Mark Fainaru-Wada and Steve Fainaru.

ESPN was involved in the documentary production for approximately fifteen months before dropping out of the project. Frontline announced the end of the partnership on August 22, 2013, and described a relationship—like those between the PBS investigative series and other news organizations—where Frontline and ESPN had "been in sync on the goals of our reporting: to present the deepest accounting so far of the league's handling of questions around the long-term impact of concussions" (Moughty, 2013). ESPN received criticism for its willingness to cave under pressure from the NFL during a lunch meeting where the league voiced "displeasure with the documentary" (Miller & Belson, 2013, p. D1) and its broadcast partner. While ESPN bailed on the partnership, Fainaru-Wada and Fainaru remained working with the film while reporting about head trauma in football for the sports network.

From the film's opening minute, it described "a decades-long battle between scientists, players, and the nation's most powerful sports league." The film picked up on *Head Games'* insightful discussion regarding contact sport and repetitive blows to the head but turned attention past sport—and even football—to focus solely on the NFL. Beyond a few similar interview participants in medical professionals and Schwartz, *League of Denial* offered Bennet Omalu's story and its centrality to connecting CTE—not concussions—with the NFL. This film traced the NFL's cover-up attempts regarding brain injuries in football and highlighted the 2009 congressional hearings. Furness (2016) explained that "*League of Denial* also constructs a critical counter-narrative of the complex and constitutive relationships between media, football and culture that actively contests the mythology of pro football cultivated through NFL Films and the league's spectacular representational strategies" (p. 56). This identification of Jhally's sport/media complex embedded within American culture implicated both media and the NFL for glorifying the sport's physicality and brutality to the detriment of human bodies but offered how media, at least in some small way, started to recognize the problems of its own role in this production.

Concussion *(2015)*

The last film included for analysis is not a documentary. Despite its cinematic Hollywood flair, *Concussion* was deemed critical for inclusion because of its role in creating a counter-narrative of the dramatization of football. The film was based on Jeanne Marie Laskas's book of the same title that spawned from an original story about Omalu for *Gentleman's Quarterly* magazine in 2009. *Concussion* runs counter to most mainstream Hollywood movies that depicted football for its pageantry, sportsmanship, and social goodwill. Instead, this two-hour, three-minute movie portrayed Omalu's fight against the NFL after his "discovery" of CTE in an American football player. The film failed to recognize that Mike Webster was not the first athlete or human being ever diagnosed (Smith & Stewart, 2016). Regardless, the film's ability to bring medical research in a digestible form to the big screen was deemed a success for raising public awareness to possibly question American obsession with football (Lau, 2016; Siegler & Wesley, 2016).

The film did a disservice to public understanding of concussions and CTE for two primary reasons. First, the movie was the story of Omalu's fight with the NFL over a decade about the validity of his findings and direct linkage between CTE (not concussions) and the NFL based on his initial published research in 2005 and subsequent research by Omalu and countless other medical researchers. For a film company, it would have been challenging to name the movie CTE or chronic traumatic encephalopathy because it is not a widely understood term in the public domain. While it was much easier to name the movie with a term that was commonly recognized (but really, not readily understood), the problem was that the movie's name misrepresents the actual story being told. Second, the name of the movie provides an association between concussions and CTE that was incorrect.

While the story was captivating at times and situated Pittsburgh as an epicenter of brain injuries in football, the film's name was one significant problem. Omalu's story is forever linked to CTE—*not* concussions. However, by positioning concussions alongside Omalu, the title clouded public understanding of what was at stake in the film and in Omalu's story. Concussions were not new to the NFL or football or contact sport when Omalu published his research. Unfortunately, CTE was not as sexy, or easily understood, by the public. Thus, the name of the film was simplified to a term more commonly and linguistically connected to sport. A second concern raised by Siegler and Wesley (2016) was that the film "deliberately" ignored the NFL safety standards for helmets implemented in 1973 and that this omission painted the NFL "as a macabre, deceptive, and dishonorable villain" (p. e157). Despite this oversight, the issue was the long-term effects of repeated blows to the head in football that caused life-long, debilitating neurological problems for the players highlighted in the film.

The film overemphasized deadly consequences related to CTE. Six more players after Webster committed suicide, and the film alluded to CTE as the cause for these deaths. Highlighting this extreme result of what was medically understood about symptoms of CTE, especially at the time of the film's portrayal, was problematic (Siegler & Wesley, 2016), especially given the knowledge gaps related to fully understanding any brain trauma in sport (Smith & Stewart, 2016). The film undoubtedly raised the ire of the NFL and did the same for some scientists who have discredited Omalu's work or the scientific validity of the film. However, *Concussion* provided an example of film's "immense power" (Lau, 2016, p. 669) to translate dense scientific findings into popular culture.

ANALYSIS

A grounded theory approach guided the film analysis. This approach was important because it allowed the authors to apply a constant comparative method (Glaser & Strauss, 1967) to better understand how films, as a social force, connected emergent themes that constructed an overall picture of what CTE looked like and how it came to be. Glaser and Strauss (1967) described grounded theory as a method best suited to study a phenomenon or event of interest. This approach is accomplished through multiple coding processes that "is concerned with generating and plausibly suggesting (but not provisionally testing) many categories, properties, and hypotheses about general problems" (p. 104). Glaser and Holton (2004) contended that grounded theory has become too broadly used and defined in qualitative research and that at its core, grounded theory must be guided by an emergent process that is collected, coded, and conceptualized through continuously written memos that allowed theoretical themes to evolve.

The authors hoped to avoid the theoretical pitfalls through a rigorous process of open and axial coding that allowed emergent themes presented by the films of CTE as a phenomenon (Strauss & Corbin, 1990). Two authors started the open coding process and viewed each film multiple times during a two-month period. Each author recorded field notes based on individual thematic analysis intended to break down and examine the films for comparative categories and topics. The authors then discussed these separate analyses, at which point the authors began axial coding. This process reconstructed the data by making connections across the identified categories that emerged during the individual coding. The intended outcome was to identify core categories and relate them to each other (Strauss & Corbin, 1990).

This in-depth coding process revealed four primary themes as apparent across all three films. These themes are discussed in the following order: (1) whistleblowers and the media, (2) science versus football, (3) humanizing the NFL player, and (4) family dynamic. Some common patterns progressed from one film to the next. Each film offered a unique perspective and provided different vantage points, but the overriding commonality was that contact sport, primarily football, must be reevaluated moving forward both for long-term sustainability and a viable need to better appreciate and understand "the brain is the last frontier" as described so eloquently and succinctly by NFL Hall of Fame quarterback Steve Young in *League of Denial*. Young was diagnosed with at least seven concussions, the last of which ended his playing career in 1999.

Like most cases of major news stories that reach the public as an availability cascade, there were two necessary ingredients that moved CTE into a constant and consistent mediated space. First, multiple sources provided significant information regarding some wrongdoing.

Second, news outlets published the information for public consumption. In the case of CTE and brain injuries in sport, this film analysis identified five primary individuals and one significant news organization who drove the story that was further developed over the years by a wide range of media members.

Whistleblowers and the Media

The five individuals who served as CTE whistleblowers against American football, specifically to the NFL, in these films were Nowinski, Omalu, Schwarz, and the Fainaru brothers. Their respective significance throughout the formative years of breaking news to the public regarding the long-term effects of brain injuries in football was paramount to unearthing an NFL cover-up that gained negative publicity akin to Big Tobacco. While Omalu published the initial findings, it was through the collective sharing of these findings that opened Pandora's box on the NFL and secondarily contact sports.

Omalu received early credit from media and scientific journals. In the films, however, he was not interviewed in *Head Games* and only received a brief mention before he became a focal point in the other two films. This omission was somewhat surprising given the long-standing connection and overlap between Nowinski and Omalu (Nowinski, 2007; Schwarz, 2007a). Instead, it was Nowinski who was first portrayed as a whistleblower in *Head Games*, primarily through his serendipitous relationship with Schwarz, who reviewed an early manuscript for Nowinski's eventual book. Schwarz explained in the film that the content of the book was good, but it was the meticulous and detailed research evident in the footnotes that made Schwarz begin investigating brain injuries in football and, subsequently, CTE.

Nowinski's link to the science of CTE and its connection to football shifted in *League of Denial* because of his individual motivation as well as through a new relationship with researchers at Boston University led by Ann McKee. The film's narrator outlined, "For Nowinski, the issue of CTE is personal. He worries he has it" (Kirk, Gilmore, & Wiser, 2013). He was described as the guy who obtained brains for research. Arguably the most significant brain that Nowinski gathered for CTE research was that of Andre Waters, who played twelve seasons between 1984 and 1995 for the Arizona Cardinals and the Philadelphia Eagles. Waters was forty-four years old when he shot himself in November 2006 in Tampa, Florida. In December, Nowinski visited with Waters's family and was granted access to his brain, which was sent to Omalu.

Omalu is often credited with naming—not discovering—CTE in an American football player that offered the first challenge to football, despite his noted lack of knowledge of the sport or the players he examined during autopsies. Despite the passing reference to him in *Head Games*,

Omalu was central to the other two films for his initial diagnosis of Webster and for repeated diagnoses over the following years. Omalu was primarily depicted through *League of Denial* and *Concussion* for his battle with the NFL over credibility. That theme was critical to Omalu and the questioning of his research that came from MTBI committee members, the NFL commissioner, and even family members of Junior Seau. The question of whether Omalu's research was groundbreaking or self-inflated also challenged his credibility.

Where Omalu had support was from journalists and their continued research and in-depth reporting about brain injuries in football. Schwarz was ahead of the pack (as commissioner Tagliabue would have liked the public to think of journalists as a collective out to get the NFL). Schwarz wrote more than one hundred articles related to brain injuries in sports for the *New York Times* between 2007 and 2011. The seminal article, when Schwarz was a freelance writer, appeared on the paper's front page and provided the public link between Nowinski and Omalu as well the paper's first reference to CTE. Schwarz's methodical reporting was later praised because he "put the issue on the agenda of lawmakers, sports leagues, and the media at large—and helped create a new debate about risk and responsibility in sports" (Marx, 2011, p. 109). Schwarz was prominently featured in both documentaries, and the *Times'* headlines for his articles were significantly discussed and portrayed in *Concussion* as critical for public knowledge that helped fuel the 2009 congressional hearings.

Schwarz led the media blitz of CTE in football, and it was the Fainaru brothers who connected the dots to position CTE squarely on the NFL through the league's constant denial of a connection between football and brain injuries. The brothers were not new to breaking stories. Steve Fainaru covered the Iraq war for the *Washington Post* beginning in 2004 and won the 2008 Pulitzer Prize for international reporting on security contractors. Before *League of Denial*, Mark Fainaru-Wada, along with fellow *San Francisco Chronicle* writer Lance Williams, broke the story in 2003 of Bay Area Laboratory Co-Operative (BALCO) and its distribution of performance-enhancing drugs to professional athletes, primarily focused on all-time home runs leader Barry Bonds. In 2006, they wrote *The Game of Shadows* that detailed the legal and federal cases involving BALCO and Bonds (Cabot, 2011). Fainaru-Wada (2011) later explained, "It is every reporter's dream to feel as if his work has an impact and elicits change" (p. 77). Their reporting, much like Schwarz's for the NFL, led to congressional hearings about steroids in baseball and began to raise public awareness about an endemic problem.

The book, *League of Denial*, and subsequent film pushed the focus of brain trauma in sport solely to the NFL. The Fainaru brothers' detailed account of Omalu's research, the NFL's attempt to damn his name, and the uncovering of medical records to discredit the NFL's published research was a remarkable example of answering journalism's primary questions: how and why. To protect its multi-billion-dollar enterprise, the NFL attempted to tear down the credibility of published research and long-form journalism. As Carey (1986) explained, "How and why are the most problematic aspects of American journalism: the dark continent and invisible landscape. Why and how are what we most want to get out of a news story and are least likely to receive or what we must in most cases supply ourselves" (p. 149). The Fainaru brothers explored the dark continent of brain injuries caused by football and provided the impetus for *League of Denial* and *Concussion* to reveal the story of whistleblowers and the collective fight for public understanding of an invisible injury that resulted in multiple unexplainable deaths.

Science vs. Football

The consistent theme of whistleblowers across the three films both clouded and confirmed why CTE in football was significant. This challenge was perpetuated by the number of scientists who were situated as experts and who spoke about CTE and/or repeated brain injuries. The desire by scientists and journalists, even if not admitted in the films, to battle the NFL empire was subtle and consistent across each of the films and throughout the research literature. The challenge became who should be the leading voice. As exemplified across these three films, there was a battle for recognition over who was driving the research (e.g., medical doctors, Nowinski) and who was reporting it.

Overall, none of the three films legitimately questioned the findings of the scientists. The films did allow for NFL-funded researchers to briefly challenge the validity. However, doctors such as Omalu and McKee were provided ample space to speak about their respective battles against the NFL and to perpetuate a scientific argument with their research about the influence of football on brain trauma. The discussion here was important for two reasons. First, the relationship between science and mass media in perpetuating public health issues has historically raised concerns about the rapid distribution of information and the impact of reduced coverage on perception of public urgency (Goodell, 1987) as exemplified in chapter 2 regarding HIV/AIDS. Second, research about brain injuries, specifically CTE, in contact sports has been skewed since the first brains were donated through a convenience sample, arguably to the greatest skewed level ever for research related to any chronic health issue that received this significant level of media attention. Since these films were released, published research started to account for the strength of selection bias and applied to a "plausible value" to estimate the prevalence of CTE. This attempt to conceptualize perceived bias provided statistical reason as a counternarrative to early and repeated concerns surrounding bias (Binney & Bachynski, 2019).

The films did their respective due diligence to articulate a story, but they are situated with a pro-science agenda against football and contact sports regarding the direct and indirect links to repeated brain trauma and long-term effects. Therefore, it was important to identify the people responsible for the films (e.g., scientists, journalists, filmmakers) who each had a stake in potential personal and financial gain based upon a story that painted the NFL in a negative light. Additionally, it exemplified a direct reflection of a public culture interested in mediated conflict. While the films did little to question any scientific validity, the scientific community has challenged whether published research has verified a direct link between football or contact sports and CTE (Hazrati et al., 2013; Randolph, 2018; Solomon, 2018; Tator, 2014). This debate between scientists, both independently and NFL funded, and football explained largely why CTE research received significant levels of media attention despite the controversial number of limited cases (Goodell, 1987).

McKee and her Boston University colleagues (e.g., Cantu, Stern) seized media—and film—attention from Omalu and Bailes as well as brains after Nowinski parted from Omalu in 2008 (Leavy, 2012). McKee also received negative attention like Omalu for her findings. Despite not being situated as a whistleblower in this analysis, McKee became the leading scientific voice against the NFL because of her work at the BU brain bank and continued published reports about the high rate of CTE in NFL postmortem brains. In *League of Denial*, journalist Jane Leavy described McKee as "a lightning rod because people see her as the woman out to destroy football as we know it. Probably the most hurtful charge that's been leveled against her is that she's crossed the line from scientist to activist." McKee's stance regarding the debate over her scientific findings was summed up in the film. Despite being questioned about sampling bias, she said, "We have still been just ridiculously successful in getting examples of this disease" and that if the greater than 99 percent rate of diagnosis was in any other brain disease, the findings would be considered extraordinary. The narrator followed, "To her, it may be the beginning of an epidemic." McKee said, "I think it's going to be a shockingly high number percentage. I'm really wondering where this stops. I'm really wondering, on some level, if every single football player doesn't have this" (Kirk et al., 2013).

This overriding sentiment among medical professionals leading CTE research was clearly articulated across all the films. However, the conflicted enjoyment of playing and watching sports was revealed by doctors, coaches, parents, and players. Despite increased knowledge of the risks of brain injuries and long-term cognitive effects, none of the three films claimed that science should earn a victory over football. Instead, the collective films made the case that mounting scientific findings must be recognized by everyone as evidence to try to limit brain injuries, especially through repetitive acts, to minimize potential harm against individual athletes.

Humanizing the NFL Player

Interestingly, the voices embroiled in the CTE debate, both in mainstream media and these films, were scientists, journalists, NFL executives, and other public officials. The glaring omission in the discussion was the players. These individuals are the often-exchanged commodity in the billion-dollar football enterprise. As Schwarz said in *League of Denial*, "They (the players) were missing time. These valuable commodities were not playing. Gee, I wonder if we (the NFL) can figure out how to keep them on the field." Sadly, the faces of CTE were most often left for secondary sources to tell their stories and guide the discussion because the primary source was dead.

From Webster to Long and Duerson to Seau, these players were the masculine heroes left to be talked about as the people who suffered from the long-term effect of brain injuries. While each film in this analysis discussed a wide variation of NFL players, their stories were situated as cautionary, concerning, and, sometimes, caustic. Webster will forever be the face of CTE. That distinction of being first was not something he strived for during his hall of fame career or as his mind spiraled out of control. As Omalu said in *Concussion*, "cardiac arrest may be how he died but not why." Webster was the unfortunate recipient of timing because his brain offered the impetus for journalists and scientists to begin asking how and why questions that produced a link between CTE and football. Additionally, these films helped to humanize these individuals to break them away from athletic accolades and introduced them as people, often troubled individuals.

The films, not surprisingly, introduced Webster and his story that extensively built off the narratives developed through historical newspaper reporting. Interestingly, Andre Waters emerged as one player who received significant attention, not necessarily for the amount of time he was discussed in the films but in being linked to when CTE hit the press and public. Waters was positioned as an ideal case study of how and why a football player could contract this degenerative brain disease. Described in every film for his hard-hitting style as a safety, Waters never played in a Pro Bowl but was good enough to stretch his career across 12 NFL seasons. He exemplified countless players, those who remain out of the limelight yet had the longevity at a high-contact position to attain numerous brain injuries.

A conflicted scene in *Concussion* provided a snapshot of the struggles facing NFL players afflicted with CTE. Waters confronted Dave Duerson, the eleven-year veteran who was a member of the famed 1985 Chicago Bears Super Bowl champions. At the time of their exchange, Duerson was part of a six-member NFL panel who considered disability claims filed by former players (Schwarz, 2011), one of which was denied for Waters (Laskas, 2009). In the movie, Waters said to Duerson, who also played safety, "You and me, we were the same, man. We were bangers, hitmen." Duerson tersely responded in a league-like response, "File the appeal." Waters continued to confront Duerson and expressed that his twelve-year career warranted something from the league to help with what he described as mental suffering. Waters said, "I'm just asking back what I gave." Duerson briefly responded, "Got a headache, see a doctor" and attempted to walk away. Waters called Duerson a "sellout" and reminisced about why they played football as kids and pleaded for Duerson's help. The next scene outlined Waters's death and funeral. Family members of both Waters and Duerson disputed the portrayal of each man in the film (Belson, 2015; Habib, 2015), but the powerful exchange encapsulated the internal battle described by athletes who have suffered with long-term cognitive effects.

While the cinematic portrayal was questioned, *Concussion* director Peter Landesman claimed it was crucial to include Duerson in the film as a metaphor for brain injuries in football. Duerson committed suicide in 2011 and left a note that asked to have his brain examined for CTE. Landesman said, "At the end of day, he (Duerson) takes his own life in the name of the disease which ravaged a lot of men that he said no to and finds himself in the ironic position of suffering from the same fate" (Dubin, 2015, para. 16). Yes, the film positioned Duerson as somehow single-handedly denying Waters, so it was important to note that Duerson was part of a committee whose votes were reportedly confidential. Regardless, this conflicted role to support the NFL's fight against brain injuries and his untimely cause of death offered a necessary juxtaposition to provide viewers with a humanizing element of the struggle related to CTE and other long-term cognitive effects.

Waters's story was explained in *Head Games* as the reason Gene Atkins, a safety with the New Orleans Saints, was evaluated by Dr. Cantu. Atkins's wife contacted Nowinski following the Waters story in the *Times*. In a frightful scene, Atkins cannot remember sequential months of the year or basic number order. Atkins served as an example of the fear family members have for an athlete who was not close to the person they were mentally before playing contact sports. This does not mean Atkins has CTE, but his story, connected to Waters, provided viewers with a sense of long-term cognitive effects suffered by former football players. The NFL's belated admission of a connection between brain trauma and cognitive effect as well as the noted $765-million concussion settlement served to couch this discussion in each film of how to repay these players, which was virtually impossible when or if brain function was lost.

Link to Big Tobacco

The films were not produced to argue against contact sports, but instead, to debate whether a player with a head injury should be allowed to return to a game, and potentially, to a sport—ever. The argument was vetted as new knowledge added to public discourse nearly every week, which produced a debate between what was known and what people should do with that new information. Scientific research about CTE in football is still in its infancy, and thus has not dissuaded people from participating despite knowledge of the direct cause of a preventable death. These same hurdles were faced by researchers who studied smoking and other environmental hazards, who were often intercepted by marketing efforts that continued to inform people about how to find information about quitting smoking rather than promoting prevention (Noar et al., 2016). One comparison between smoking and CTE centered on whether this developing scientific research about brain injuries in sport would influence public perception or lead to willingness to not participate.

Beyond knowledge and information, however, the films highlighted a mediated conflict between science and football that reached public prominence because of a cover-up and falsification of research, which sounded eerily similar to Big Tobacco in the 1950s. This conflict painted the NFL as a villain with deliberate interest in the outcome of what science was finding related to brain injuries. The most damning moment for the NFL was the 2009 congressional hearings. The NFL has a history with Congress, but nothing quite like this (Drysdale, 2013; Smith, 2013), and the films found this poignant moment as necessary to include in the story.

Each of the three films provided prominent space for a direct quote from Linda Sanchez. The California member of the United States House of Representatives since 2003 said to commissioner Goodell in 2009, "the NFL sort of reminds me of the tobacco companies, pre-90s, when they kept saying, 'no, there's no link between smoking and damage to your health or ill health effect.'" When named commissioner in 2006, Goodell was handed a potential firestorm that linked head injuries to football. The Big Tobacco/NFL comparison started before Sanchez's quote, but this congressional bomb was one of the gravest public relations nightmares for the NFL. As Fainaru-Wada said in *League of Denial*, "The last thing the league wanted to be dealing with in that moment was the analogy to Big Tobacco. There's nobody in America that doesn't know what that means. That means denial" (Kirk et al., 2013). Remember, it was commissioner Tagliabue who was in charge during the misconstrued medical research produced by the MTBI Committee. However, Goodell was the target under the greatest scrutiny who faced public backlash on the NFL's behalf (Smith, 2013).

In *Concussion*, Omalu was positioned in a fight against one of America's most powerful—and popular—organizations. His lasting argument was for the NFL to "tell the truth," which the league had little interest in admitting to or paying out. Sanchez and several other congressional members, despite limited input from Omalu or admission from the NFL, produced a public condemnation of the league. Each film readily included it in the story of brain injuries that instantly generated a cause-and-effect link between football and brain injuries, largely in conjunction with CTE. It was nearly seven years between Omalu's diagnosis of CTE in 2002 and the congressional hearings involving Sanchez. Ironically, after another seven-year stretch and following the three films, the NFL publicly acknowledged a link between football and CTE (Armour, 2016; Campbell & Walker, 2016). Regardless of the time involved between these seminal moments, it was the intersection of Congress, the NFL, and, at a closer-than-expected distance, Big Tobacco (Schwarz et al., 2016) that this reached a level of public outcry and frustration to attain significant placement in each film.

Each film provided some context for the link between tobacco and football, regarding their parallel strategies of denial of causation. The MTBI Committee and the fourteen-part series published in *Neurosurgery* was outlined to discuss Pellman's medical training as a rheumatologist with no experience in neurology. This presentation helped each film provide viewers with insight into the fraudulent construction of the MTBI Committee from the outset. The films fell short since they could have further compared the use of the TIRC by Big Tobacco to construct favorable medical findings, which was the function of the MTBI Committee. Ira Casson was portrayed as a villain connected to his televised denial on HBO's *Real Sports* in 2009, where he responded "no" to four consecutive questions of whether football related to a variety of degenerative neurological disorders. Casson's response was used in the films and by Sanchez during the congressional hearings. This contextual parallel to Big Tobacco provided why each of these films positioned the NFL in a negative light because of a long-standing tradition of denial and use of political clout involved with medical research to perpetuate the league's agenda and financial bottom line (Bachynski & Goldberg, 2018).

Family Dynamic

The final theme that emerged was the impact of CTE on families. While secondarily connected to football, the ability of each film to show how CTE affected extended families provided the best lens to see its effect. Thus, the films juxtaposed several social forces involved in athletic participation that weighed the desire for families to have their children succeed in sports versus the lasting impact of head injuries on the athletes who suffer them but also the parents, spouses, children, and medical doctors who are left to deal with the lasting impact. *Head Games*'s opening scene witnessed a youth football game where the coach positioned his team in a David-vs.-Goliath game where violence would have to win out. The coach explained to his players, "This is your rock, your helmet." This insinuated a need to use the helmet as a defense mechanism or to inflict pain, which has perpetuated as a masculine ideal in the sport for more than a century. Underlying this statement shielded by sports clichés (e.g., using sports to overcome, defeat the odds, level the playing field), these films outlined a sad truth of sport: the better an athlete performed usually equaled a longer-than-likely playing career and a greater risk for long-term brain injuries.

People like Pam and Garrett Webster, Lisa McHale, Tom Thomas, Katherine Brealey, Sydney and Tyler Seau each played a role in these films and offered varying accounts of suffering. They were the family members of players who died and were left to try to make sense of why the men they knew killed themselves. Then people like Keith Primeau, Steve Young, Cindy Parlow Cone, and Roger Staubach offered examples of the athletes who reached the peak of their respective sport and suffered varying levels of memory loss related to repeated head injuries, whether documented or unknown. They have children or coached youth sports and grappled with the idea of whether they should play sports and how to deal with potential brain injuries. Additionally, parents of youth athletes personified the tension produced by the family dynamic. They had children who played soccer, football, and hockey among other sports who suffered concussions. Each one questioned when they should consider removing their child from a given sport but admitted that selfishly they enjoyed watching their kids succeed on the field or ice and could not bring themselves to stop their dream of playing professional sports. Lastly, there were the scientists who saw the lasting effects daily, both in living patients and deceased brains. Omalu's wife, Prema Mutiso, was characterized in *Concussion* for helping Omalu cope with the embroiled battle for his reputation against the NFL.

These scientists relied on their findings to make a case against athletic participation in contact sports, especially for children. The overarching message was that all people are granted one brain during their life and it should be treated as the most valuable commodity they could ever possess. McKee was asked hypothetically in *League of Denial* if she had children who were eight, ten, or twelve years old, would she allow them the play football. Her response was that they would not play football "because the way football is being played currently, that I've seen, it's dangerous. It's dangerous. It could impact their long-term mental health. You only get one brain. The thing you want your kids to do, most of all, is succeed in life and be everything they can be." Douglas Smith, director for the Center for Brain Injury and Repair at the University of Pennsylvania, said toward the end of *Head Games*, if he sustained a brain injury in sport, he would wait fifty years to return to the sport. His simple rationale: "That's my brain. If you get hit again, you're going down another notch. If you like how quickly you can think now, like who you are, and that you can get jokes quickly. What if that went away? For me, that's enough of a risk to just say no."

ADVANCING CTE THROUGH FILM

It is necessary to recognize that each film provided unique and differing perspectives, but the connection was that each was guided by Ricketson's (2016) call for slow journalism over time that allowed a story to evolve and started to connect the dots. Each film framed a certain agenda through the primary interviewees. However, the common thread across each story was how to battle against brain injuries in sport and to position the athlete and their respective long-term safety at the forefront, regardless of age, gender, or level of sport. Reflecting on the analogy that the brain is the last frontier for science, these films allowed time to process long-term effects often connected to what players, coaches, and media simplify as short-term brain injuries (e.g., concussions).

Situated within a journalistic context, the order of these three films flowed like the historically rooted inverted pyramid writing style. By starting with the who, what, when, where, why, and how, viewers received general information before drilling down in greater detail. *Head Games* provided the overview of brain injuries in sport and the awareness needed to begin the conversation. *League of Denial* purported the most significant problem for brain injuries in sport and related it to football. *Concussion* focused on the person who broke the news. Therefore, when viewing these three films, it should be considered to watch them in a linear fashion. Approaching these films in chronological order offered a wonderful contextualization of the evolution and manifestation of CTE guided by the slow news approach of long-form journalism that centered the primary focus of brain injuries caused by football.

Film further perpetuated the media narrative constructed by newspapers that CTE was a football problem and attempted to challenge its masculine hold on contact sport. For example, Furness (2016) explained that *League of Denial* served to oppose "the dominant discourses that normalize and naturalize violence" (Furness, 2016, p. 56) previously rooted in a system where "players were taught to deny pain" (Sabo & Panepinto, 1990, p. 123). Instead, the films added expert context in their respective use of scientists to drive the conversation and, ultimately, problematize masculinity. However, as the next chapter outlines, the media framing through newspapers and film over more than a decade raised important questions about risk of long-term effect of brain injuries for boys and men playing American football, and in the process, excluded other at-risk groups that reified the hold of hegemonic masculinity on what is often perceived as newsworthy.

EIGHT

It's a "Guy Thing"

Mediated Misconceptions

CTE, from a media perspective, has not been equitable in sport. The newspaper stories and films included in this book nearly eliminated female-specific sports from any discourse connected to CTE. Newspapers did allow some space for sports such as hockey and soccer that do include female participants. However, when considering who participates professionally in these sports, which receive significant media exposure, hockey and soccer—with isolated exceptions for the World Cup—are still considered masculine sporting spaces. Fink (2015) explained that critical media scholars have suggested "this differential treatment by the sport media is a conscious effort to maintain male power and privilege" (p. 337). In the construction of CTE, media supported Fink's assertion and missed nearly twenty at-risk sports for concussions and other brain injuries that have been identified as a precursor to CTE and thus should have space in the conversation about risks of CTE.

Built largely on a cascade of published scientific research, media discourse in the twenty-first century, instead, constructed CTE as a *football* epidemic. Over the course of CTE as a developing story and thinking back to how HIV/AIDS was framed by media in its early stage as a deviant result of homosexuality or drug use, CTE witnessed strikingly similar positioning connected to an atypical group. Both diseases were perceived to be a result of an individual's continued participation in an at-risk activity. It was somewhat ironic to see so many parallels between how media framed two diseases across such disparate groups on opposite sides of the masculinity scale. Ultimately, CTE was framed as a diagnosis for men.

As of January 2019, CTE has not been diagnosed in a female athlete. In fact, only two cases of CTE (or at least retroactively labeled) have been diagnosed—ever—in a female. A 1990 published report described a domestic violence victim in Britain who showed punch-drunk symptoms (Roberts et al., 1990). Even that case was only tangentially connected based on scientific advances and speculation that the diagnosis would now be CTE. One year later, the second published case was identified in an autism patient who suffered myriad forms of self-injury. The authors noted tangles in unexpected parts of her brain and connected it to similar findings in boxers and soccer players with repeated head trauma (Hof, Knabe, Bovier, & Bouras, 1991). Thus, in nearly three decades since, nothing else connected women and CTE.

This is partially explained because the potential for CTE diagnosis has been limited to available brains. In 2016, Brandi Chastain announced a pledge to donate her brain to the Concussion Legacy Foundation when she dies. The former star of the 1999 U.S. Women's World Cup championship soccer team was one of the first female athletes to make that pledge. A 2016 story in the *Washington Post* identified how rare a female brain has been for examination. Of the 307 brains donated to the foundation at BU's CTE Center, only four were women compared to more than two hundred from former football players (Maese, 2016). Thus, the dataset has been severely skewed toward men, which perpetuated the strengthening force of CTE as an availability cascade that media consistently linked to American football. McKee was quoted in the story, "We currently know so little about how gender influences outcome after trauma" (Maese, 2016, para. 7). However, research showed the potential, if brains become available, both for the study of gender and other sports (Eme, Gilbertson, & Oehler, 2013; Keene, Latimer, Steele, & MacDonald, 2018).

Brain injuries and their symptoms, as well as short- and long-term effects have been widely addressed concerning professional athletes, especially those in the NFL. As discussed throughout this book, the NFL has remained the most popular American sport despite any threat of perceived, or actual, risk of playing football. While football deserved a significant space in the discussion about brain injuries in sport, due largely to its violent nature, other sports such as basketball, hockey, soccer, and lacrosse should not be ignored. Cantu and Hyman (2012) included these sports among thirteen highlighted as *at-risk* for brain injuries. Furthermore, these sports have gained traction among young adults and youth leagues through increased participation and have contributed to the growing problem of brain trauma in sport (Bodenner, 2016; Ortiz, 2016; Otero, 2015).

Focusing media attention on football (with hockey and boxing occasionally linked as collision sports) left little opportunity to explore the full scope of brain injury for athletes across all sports, especially in considering gender differences. This was problematic because parents could get a false sense that a non-collision sport could be less likely to lead to brain trauma. Instead, research showed child participation in any sport, regardless of level of contact, can lead to a concussion (Covassin, Savage, Bretzin, & Fox, 2018; Tanveer, Zecavati, Delasobera, & Oyegbile, 2017).

Rather than contribute to the narrative that only collision and contact sports pose a threat to the safety and well-being of youth athletes, differences in brain injuries across sport and gender expand the conversation beyond the NFL as well as to implicate media as part of the problem. CTE is the primary focus of this book, and the authors recognize that it is a likely outcome of repetitive brain injuries regardless of whether they were diagnosed or not. However, this chapter includes a significant discussion connected to concussions, which this research also recognizes as a significantly connected (albeit not the only) brain injury to CTE. The reason to include concussions in the discussion is to highlight the mounting scientific research that should be explained in any reporting of CTE, which could produce a more visible picture of gender risks than the nearly extinct female category currently available in CTE research and media presence.

RISK IN ALL SPORTS

During the 2016–2017 school year, approximately eight million high school boys and girls played sports on a school-sponsored team in the United States. The most popular sports among this group were football and soccer, which increased the concern of concussion risks among parents in those sports (Flanagan, 2017). Meanwhile, sports like basketball, ice hockey, and wrestling also had high school–aged athletes at risk for head injury. For example, one study found that boys who participated in wrestling sustained concussions at a rate of 6 percent ("Football not only," 2012). Though this number may seem small, it indicated a need to recognize that football and soccer were not the only contact sports where young athletes may be concussed. Cantu and Hyman (2012) understood that when they recognized wrestling as a sport that posed a high risk of catastrophic brain injuries. Regardless of the sport played, common misconceptions suggested that coaches, parents, players, and administrators must understand and accept the risk that exists for *any* sport in which a child participated (Harmon et al., 2013).

As this book has outlined, media have the significant space and perceived authority to shape public understanding by how they frame information. In the process, media can skew the conversation away from who could be at risk of brain injuries in sport. A report from *Safe Kids Worldwide* identified concussions as the fourth most common injury among youth athletes that resulted in an emergency room visit in 2012 ("Game changer," 2013). Athletes in that report were taken to the emergency room primarily for injuries related to sprains and strains, fractures, and contusions. While bodily injury can be significant and life-threatening, in most cases the body can heal and be mended because of the knowledge that exists toward repairing injuries with obvious outward, physical signs. However, the alarming statistic for concussions was that kids between ages twelve and fifteen accounted for 47 percent of those cases ("Game changer," 2013). Based on these numbers, protecting a child's brain should be the top priority, especially since it has not fully developed until their twenties and, thus, is disproportionately at greater risk of injury during adolescence when compared to the rest of the body (Arain et al., 2013).

Football is well documented as a leading cause of aggregate concussions in sport. The *Safe Kids* study supported the conclusion that football accounts for 35 percent of the documented 163,670 concussions in emergency room visits. However, basketball (20 percent), soccer (15 percent), and baseball/softball (13 percent) each accounted for a substantial proportion of the total documented cases (Healy, 2013). Deeper in the findings, ice hockey resulted in the fewest number of total injuries but the highest percentage of concussions (31 percent) in the sport. Wrestling was (14 percent) second, followed by American football and soccer each at 13 percent ("Game changer," 2013). It was important to note these findings were only emergency visits, so these are only part of the total picture of brain injuries in youth sport (Healy, 2013). Therefore, if repeated hits to the head often result in concussions and can be a cause of CTE, then these numbers alone identify a nearly invisible at-risk population that media have excluded in a disproportionate number of news stories.

In a study of pediatric concussions in the Washington, D.C., area, nineteen sports resulted in concussions that were documented and treated between 2010 and 2016. This study included sports widely discussed as contact sports (e.g., football, lacrosse, rugby) but also identified instances, sometimes at high rates, in non-contact sports (e.g., cheerleading, swimming, volleyball) (Tanveer et al., 2017). As a popular thought in media reports, soccer is argued beyond football as "probably the sport that has the most [concussions], because they tend to collide heads while running for the ball. It's very contact heavy" (Ortiz, 2016, para. 2). This observation by an athletic trainer was supported by scientific research that indicated an increase in concussions in soccer with the largest number of concussions from athlete-to-athlete contact, followed by heading the ball, which has been a well-publicized topic of debate for the long-term safety of soccer (Comstock, Currie, & Pierpoint, 2015). However, lacrosse was identified as a cause of more concussions, with a greater risk in a game than in practice (Reynolds et al., 2016; Tanveer et al., 2017).

For years, there was an idea that only if children engaged in contact sports, they faced the greatest risk of sustaining a potential long-term brain injury (Daugherty & Sarmiento, 2018), possibly started by a concussion. However, a child can suffer a brain injury engaging in many activities that are often incorrectly considered safe (i.e., female, non-collision) such as cheerleading, gymnastics, or volleyball. For example, cheerleading witnessed a nearly 300 percent increase in pediatric head injuries between 2001 and 2012 (Naiyer, Chounthirath, & Smith, 2017). Cheerleaders often participate in group stunting routines and individual gymnastics (via tumbling), which present various opportunities for head injuries and are considered the greatest risk in the sport (Salamon, 2015). Additionally, synchronized swimming has an alarmingly high rate of concussions because of the choreographed routines that require swimmers to work in unison (Cantu & Hyman, 2012). Thus, sports considered non-contact have proved to be just as risky as contact sports for short- and long-term brain injuries.

Two reasons are offered to consider for a lack of insight into this growing trend of misinformation. First, young athletes have not recognized whether they have a concussion because they were not properly educated about the signs of concussions or other brain-related trauma (Knollman-Porter, Brown, & Flynn, 2018; Wallace, Covassin, Nogle, Gould, & Kovan, 2017). A decrease in certified athletic trainers at the high school level has been one likely cause for lack of understanding. This loss of experienced adults on the sidelines has been attributed to budget restrictions and lack of proximity to medical facilities and that has impacted a decrease in the number of properly diagnosed head injuries (Kroshus, Rivara, Whitlock, Herring, & Chrisman, 2017; Mazerolle, Raso, Pagnotta, Stearns, & Casa, 2015). However, one study found that while access to an athletic trainer did increase an athlete's knowledge, it did not increase willingness to report a head injury (Wallace et al., 2017).

This unwillingness led to the second consideration that athletes hide an injury to continue playing as a reflection of the masculine ideology of the pain principle (Sabo, 2009). One study identified that female college athletes were more willing than male athletes to identify symptoms related to a concussion and that the male athletes were more willing to risk—and hide—injury for winning (Kroshus, Baugh, Stein, Austin, & Calzo, 2017). Thus, the male athletes fit into the masculine ideology embedded in American contact sport that to play through pain is often glorified by media and "produced as part of the orthodox notions of commitment to sport and victory" (Anderson & Kian, 2012, p. 155). However, the study found no difference in likelihood to sit out from competition because of the potential risk from a known injury. Therefore, females were also willing to participate in some risk-taking behaviors (Kroshus et al., 2017). These findings offered interesting insight into a willingness to play through risk. Further exploration about gender differences was needed to offer more context within the conversation surrounding issues of brain injuries in sport.

GENDER MATTERS

Females share equal risks of brain injury to their male counterparts, yet discussions surrounding the impact on this group are often buried in media discourse, due to the focus on concussions in male-dominated sports such as football. As this injury risk for female athletes has increased through more participation, more information has become available to address the severity of traumatic brain injuries, specifically those like concussions, and their impact on overall social, athletic, and academic well-being (Knollman-Porter et al., 2018; Harmon et al., 2013). As this research continues to grow, learning that, for example, cheerleading can lead to brain injuries—which is more often labeled an activity, rather than a sport—highlights the importance for parents, teachers, coaches, and participants to acknowledge these injuries may result from participation. In the *Safe Kids* research, cheerleading produced the sixth-most emergency room visits among the fourteen youth sports included in their study ("Game changer," 2013). Bringing this knowledge to light should signal a need to shift the conversation about mild traumatic brain injuries, but unfortunately, as Sabo (2009) explained, despite these findings that offer "public health implications" for all athletes, "there has been no major groundswell to change [the culture of] *men's* sports" (p. 150). Sadly, that would be necessary for any sweeping change, but "the patterns of economic incentive and exploitation" (Sabo, 2009, p. 150) are what hinder the process. Subsequently, the discourse continues to overwhelmingly focus on football, and the identification of the *male* athlete as at-risk (Aschwanden, 2016).

Contrastingly, research has indicated that females *are at greater risk* than males for brain injuries when comparing similar sports played by both groups, including basketball, lacrosse, hockey, soccer, and baseball/softball (Cantu & Hyman, 2012; Comstock et al., 2015; Covassin, Moran, & Elbin, 2016; Tanveer et al., 2017). Much of this research, however, focused on the sports that caused injury, rather than the aftermath in managing symptoms and recovering time. These can be physically and psychologically different based on gender. For example, female athletes have experienced higher levels of symptoms following concussions than their male counterparts (Covassin et al., 2018; Tanveer et al., 2017). These findings suggest a possible chink in the masculine armor of sport regarding brain injuries, at least in the medical literature, that have been selectively discussed in mainstream media (Anzidei, 2018; Bogage, 2017; Fox, 2018; Healy, 2013; Kwon, 2017), albeit in isolated stories that do not offer much context over time.

Instead, a cultural and ideological shift in the journalistic process is necessary to increase overall media attention for female athletics beyond tennis as well as biennial (e.g., Olympics) and quadrennial (e.g., World Cup) competitions (Bell & Coche, 2018). This will take time considering media continue to "portray the dominant images or symbolic representations of American society" (Kane, 1988, p. 89) identified more than three decades ago. Even more important than just closing the gender gap in overall coverage of sport, issues such as brain injuries must be an impetus for change for more inclusive reporting of girls and women to ensure this vulnerable demographic is studied and therefore educated about the consequences associated with mTBI as well as avoid media tropes that position female sports as inferior that require less rigorous attention (Whiteside & Hardin, 2011). Yet, by excluding them from consistent coverage—essentially silencing them—keeps them out of public discourse surrounding brain injuries while maintaining their position of greater risk.

MEDIATING CHANGE

One area where media has engaged in reporting on brain injuries at the youth level has been with equipment and rule changes. Proper tackling techniques and minimal use of helmets in practice have been couched in football discourse. Heading in soccer has received substantial coverage grounded in science as the second-leading cause of concussions in the sport (Comstock et al., 2015). Calls to eliminate both tackling in youth football and heading in youth soccer dominated the conversation as groups weighed in on both sides about the inherent and unexpected consequences (Draper, 2015; Fainaru-Wada, 2017; Omalu, 2015). This media attention generated responses from medical professionals who explained how these decisions fueled calls to ban sports entirely, which they debated can lead to greater risk of decreased physical activity (Calderwood, Murray, & Stewart, 2016; MacDonald & Myer, 2017). Also, this call to action created public debate that challenges the normative, masculine culture of American sport (Bell & Sanderson, 2016).

Three sports (lacrosse, field hockey, cheerleading) offer brief examples of how rules and safety are affected by the gendered version of sport. A research study of 375 observed concussions identified women's lacrosse with the second-highest incident rate of concussions, trailing only football (Marshall, Guskiewicz, Shankar, McCrea, & Cantu, 2015; Halley, 2015). The high rate of concussions in women's lacrosse was explained as the result of collisions with equipment like a player's stick, not other players (Halley, 2015). Unlike men's lacrosse where a helmet was a required piece of equipment, the goalie in women's lacrosse may be the only player to wear a helmet, since headgear was optional in the women's game. Headgear was a somewhat divisive subject in the lacrosse community, as high schools looked to change the "optional" policy. For example, high schools governed by the Public Schools Athletic League (PSAL) in New York City required headgear for the 2017 season (Pennington, 2017). However, at the collegiate level, there was pushback regarding mandatory headgear, as some coaches feared it would lead to a merging of the rules, thus transforming the women's game to mirror the men, specifically the physicality inherently present in the men's game (Pennington, 2017). Currently, headgear has remained optional, but those women and girls who choose to wear it must meet the standards outlined by the U.S. Lacrosse organization.

Field hockey is a "female only" sport in the United States, and cheerleading is widely perceived as one, despite participation from high school boys and college men. In the research study of Washington, D.C., pediatric concussions, cheerleading ranked fourth and field hockey was fifth in number of concussions, trailing only football and the combined total of concussions for lacrosse and soccer across gender (Tanveer et al., 2017). Field hockey players suffered a similar risk as their female lacrosse counterparts caused by a lack of required protective equipment. In a study of college field hockey, concussions accounted for 42.8 percent of all reported injuries to the head, face, or eye. Contact with another player was the leading cause of concussion, which was surprising given the sport's essential nature as noncontact (Gardner, 2015). While cheerleading ranked fourth in total concussions in the D.C. study across all sports, regardless of gender, it accounted for the highest percentage (n = 39, 21.5 percent) of total concussions suffered by girls (Tanveer et al., 2017). The American Academy of Pediatrics and the American Medical Association each have recommended to designate cheerleading as a sport, instead of an activity. However, the NCAA and the NFHS have not followed those recommendations. As a result, cheerleading does not receive the same benefits as other sanctioned sports, such as access to athletic trainers and certified coaches and inclusions in injury surveillance systems (Naiyer et al., 2017). Instead, individual states are left to decide the proper protocol for cheerleading injuries.

These scientific findings highlight a significant concern for brain injuries in female sports that received little-to-no media attention. Again, these stories are framed by media—through near omission—as inconsequential for public knowledge. When media has decided to report on medical findings about concussions in female sports, it focused on gender-specific differences or effects, including the impact of concussions on menstrual cycles (Emanuel, 2017). Even when publishing stories that indicated females received more concussion than males, news outlets felt necessary to include other research that proposed because women have "smaller necks" they lack the strength necessary to "absorb shock" (Kwon, 2017, para. 7). Additionally, it has been suggested that the size of the ball, compared to the size of a girl's neck, endangers them even more (Boggs, 2017). None of these media stories discussed protective equipment or rules focused on safety. Rather, they focused on gender-specific "concerns" related to concussions without assessing or critiquing dominant ideologies embedded in sport and media as the issue.

UNCONVENTIONAL ALTERNATIVES

Return-to-play guidelines have been in place across all fifty states and D.C. since 2014. However, those rules were implemented to manage a player *after an initial injury* had already occurred. Additionally, the scales used to determine when a player is deemed fit to return to athletic competition are varied (Albicini & McKinlay, 2018). As identified in the scientific research throughout this book, the number of brain injuries in sport, regardless of gender, continued to climb over the past decade. This has been attributed to greater awareness of concussions both in medicine and media but has had some adverse effects regarding concern and confusion among parents about long-term risk (Daugherty & Sarmiento, 2018; Saffary et al., 2012). Further confusion has been promulgated by media that do not inform the audience that risk can only be removed if the potential for impact to the brain is eliminated from sport (Ventresca, 2018).

As a result, participation rates in common youth sports is on the decline due to a concern of injury and competition (Johnson, 2016). As states continue to work toward creating and tweaking regulations and guidelines to protect children, finding alternative physical activity (e.g., rock climbing, fencing) for young adults has been suggested by journalists as a way to decrease risk (Cech, 2015; Ramsey, 2017). Additionally, participating in alternative opportunities could remove socialized pressure and financial burden associated with highly competitive youth sports. These activities have been suggested as a safe alternative, but as Cantu and Hyman (2012) explained, "There probably isn't a sport played by children that is concussion-proof" (p. 52). Therefore, parents must still acknowledge that injury is inherent in any sport or activity in which a child participates.

Minimizing pressure of having to play in a highly competitive sport has been ascribed several benefits. Children who participate in an alternative sport have found that they can understand who they are, and that physical activity can be fun if it aligns with their interests (Cech, 2015). Another factor that may determine whether a child participates in a traditional sport is the overall cost, especially in sports that require several pieces of equipment (e.g., helmets, padding, sticks) or significant travel through club-level teams. The equipment not only increases cost but also risk as scientific research has outlined equipment as a significant cause of head injuries. Barone (2017) reported that families, on average, spent $2,300 annually on their children to participate in sports. A survey found that some parents spend that much per month, resulting in a cost of around $24,000 per year on sports alone (Shell, 2017). This price seems minor compared to the $60,000 one family spent on practice at renowned golf facilities or to participate in specialized events, which present extreme examples. The survey indicated 63 percent of families spend between $100 and $499 monthly while 19 percent shell out $1,000 or more (Shell, 2017). In making decisions about whether to invest in elite sports, and thus paying for risk, parents must realize how the cost of participation rarely results in future earning potential through professional sport and should weigh the physical and social benefits against the cost.

Journalists have produced stories to address benefits of alternative sport-related activities. Cech (2015) followed several families whose children partake in rock climbing and badminton. A mother emphasized that allowing her child to rock climb has led to an increase in his confidence, and even committed to driving him an hour away from their home for lessons twice a week. While these parents admitted there was risk involved in these activities, they were comfortable with allowing their child to participate because they cited benefits like sportsmanship, confidence, and personal growth (Cech, 2015).

Ramsey (2017) introduced fencing as an alternate sport that has reached some African-American communities, which would be considered nontraditional and uncommon for that demographic. Parents suggested their children enjoyed the sport because of its history, critical thinking skills, and athleticism. Furthermore, one father, a former football player and the newspaper's publisher, made it clear his boys would not be allowed to play football "because of the brain trauma that can occur" (Ramsey, 2017, para. 3). Although this outlook may not be shared by all parents, these stories highlighted ways young adults have participated in active lifestyles without putting their brains at risk. It must be noted, however, that these events still cost parents money for their children to participate and can result in elite competitions, which could reshape to perceived level of risk.

CALL FOR A CULTURE SHIFT

These examples hint at a slight shift toward unconventional sports compared to the more popular and traditional contact and non-contact sports. However, unless media completely revolt in reporting on those traditional sports, it is necessary to situate the power of this influential industry to share stories of the growing amount of scientific research that is important to the safety of all sport participants. Additionally, media must become a more active and critical voice in recognizing brain injuries in sport as an epidemic that affects everyone, not just the mediated celebrities on the football field. This will require a change in media and fan culture that celebrates violence—and thus, masculinity—in sport (Foote et al., 2017; Ventresca, 2018) that should, instead, work to recognize risk and better educate the public about these inherent risks rather than reify socialized myths.

Knowing that women and girls receive inferior media coverage is problematic, as the opportunity to share scientific knowledge related to brain injuries, beyond the popularized concussion, has been limited, and at times, non-existent. Research findings highlight gender differences, including physical makeup, availability of equipment, and longer recovery time (Aschwanden, 2016; Boggs, 2017; Kwon, 2017). Therefore, brain injuries in sport do not adhere to a one-size-fits-all diagnosis (Albicini & McKinlay, 2018), and therefore, should be mediated differently. Thus, it is imperative that media increase their coverage of these critical issues to understand and discuss inherent differences in risk, recognition, and treatment. This would challenge a sports ethos that influences how athletes are willing to report and maintain treatment of brain injuries (Kroshus et al., 2017). This could further help educate the public (e.g., coaches, players, parents) about who has been susceptible to brain injuries as well as how and why that could influence overall well-being. The role of media as a conduit of public knowledge could be vital since Daugherty and Serminto (2018) identified "little educational information available to parents of youth athletes" surrounding CTE.

As evident in this chapter, there is much more that media can do—or should have done—so that equal concern, specifically for the brains, of all athletic participants maintain a consistent place in public discourse. By continuing to track and analyze data focused on girls and women, scientific researchers have valuable insight to determine how to best protect this vulnerable population of athletes. Until that research is presented through various media outlets and made available for general knowledge, parents, coaches, and athletes are left to educate themselves about concussion laws and guidelines that have been established to protect and educate those involved in sport and physical activity. Additionally, it is important to note that most sport participants are not treated with similar medical attention and long-term concern afforded to professional and elite-level college athletes. Therefore, it is incumbent upon those groups to drive funding to study the issue of brain injuries since it most affects their future labor pool.

Much like the influential research from Guskiewicz et al. (2000, 2003, 2005, 2007) at the high school and college levels that widely impacted professional sports, the NCAA and the Department of Defense (DoD) started a $30-million study of college athletes and concussions in 2014. A statement by Robin Harris, the Ivy League's executive director who is not involved with this specific study but has a vested interest in the findings, explained the rationale for such a significant study one year before it was commissioned. He said, "We recognized all along that concussions are an issue that need to be addressed whenever they happen. It's not about the sport, it's about concussions any time. . . . I know there's more conversation, as I'm sitting on the sideline at my daughter's soccer game" (Grasgreen, 2013, para. 6). The preliminary findings of the NCAA/DoD study identified that the research participants represent a "large, racially and socio-economically diverse cohort of male and female college athletes" (Katz, Kudela, Harezlak, McCrea, McAllister, & Broglio, 2018). The initial findings are largely unpublished, but it is the recognition of a breadth and depth of participants in the study that gives hope for more diverse reporting of all groups by media when the findings are prepared for public consumption about the effect of brain injuries in sport.

NINE

CTE and the NFL

Forever United

On March 14, 2016, the congressional House Energy and Commerce Subcommittee on Oversight and Investigations hosted a roundtable forum about concussions in sport. Rep. Tim Murphy opened the meeting with the substantiation that the meeting was not a formal hearing and, thus, was not considered sworn testimony before Congress. However, he asserted his assumption that because the panelists were all trained medical professionals that they would tell the truth, regardless of an oath. In an opening statement, Murphy outlined the rise of public dialogue around concussions in sport that was gaining steam after the "new and provocative" *Concussion* movie released just three months earlier ("Concussion research," 2016).

Until this March afternoon, the NFL continued to rely on its own ethically questionable research to deny that CTE was a problem, even though research from renowned neurosurgeons, neurologists, pathologists, and a multitude of other scientists had documented the foreseeable risks associated with repeated blows to the head and long-term cognitive impairment (Kain, 2009; National Football League, 2007). Even as recent as five weeks before this congressional gathering, commissioner Goodell was cited in numerous media reports for a statement made at his annual press conference two days before Super Bowl 50. When addressing the hazardous risk of playing football, Goodell said, "There are risks in life. There are risks sitting on a couch." This response received heavy, and understandable, criticism from media and family members of athletes who had been diagnosed with CTE (Campbell, 2016; Jenkins, 2016), epitomizing the continuous use of bad examples in trying to defend a link between football and risk (not guarantee) of brain injury. Therefore, as a shock to many, at the congressional forum, the NFL made its first public statement shifting its views on CTE, following years of practicing its artful craft to manufacture doubt akin to Big Tobacco years earlier (Belson & Schwarz, 2016; Goldberg, 2013; Michaels, 2008; Paolini, 2019).

Jeff Miller, the NFL's senior vice president of health and safety policy, represented the league at the congressional hearing. As he reminded the subcommittee members, he is also not a medical expert. He holds a law degree from the University of Chicago. Approximately twenty minutes into the session, Rep. Jan Schakowsky provided a summary report of documented NFL cover-up over the years and asked what she claimed should be a "yes or no" question to Ann McKee and Miller. Schakowsky asked, "Do you think there is a link between football and degenerative brain disorders like CTE?" McKee responded, "I unequivocally think there's a link between playing football and CTE" and offered data to support her claim. Schakowsky then asked, "Mr. Miller, do you think there is a link between football and degenerative brain disorders like CTE?" Miller responded, "Well, Dr. McKee's research certainly shows that a number of retired NFL players were diagnosed with CTE, so there, the answer to that question is certainly yes, but there's also a number of questions that come with that" ("Concussion research," 2016). With that short statement, the NFL admitted what media, scientists, family members, and football players saddled with debilitating brain injuries waited years to hear.

This chapter offers some concluding thoughts about the relationship between CTE and the NFL. First, the rise of CTE in public discourse is outlined for its position as an availability cascade alongside the NFL's scientific responses. Second, media framing of CTE connected to the NFL is discussed parallel with HIV/AIDS and Big Tobacco as global epidemics. Third, the impact of CTE on media representation of the NFL is contextualized within masculine ideology that has shifted incrementally toward a call for cultural change to focus on safety but avoid elimination. Finally, this chapter discusses the future of CTE within media discourse, followed by opportunities for future research in this area.

THE AVAILABILITY CASCADE OF CTE AND THE NFL

Media has a unique relationship with CTE that helped construct the disease's prominent place in the public sphere, despite claims of media sensationalism by some scientists amid this rapidly increasing flurry of attention (Baugh, Robbins, Stern, & McKee, 2014; Granier et al., 2011; Wortzel, 2014). Considered only as a purveyor of information, media performed its duty to inform the public of a growing health concern through its repeated coverage of each new scientific publication. However, media circulated information freely about CTE that was invariably interwoven with concussions as well as emphasized specific findings in medical studies to shine focus on the NFL and few other potential recipients of CTE diagnoses. This process diluted and distorted understanding of CTE—what it is, how it is diagnosed, who is at risk, and how to look for it. Media discourse of CTE teetered between awareness and confusion, sometimes simultaneously. However, through this mediated hyper focus, CTE witnessed "a 21st-century transformation" (Solomon & Sills, 2014, p. 26) fueled by congressional hearings, questions surrounding youth safety in contact sports, litigation, increased scientific findings, and public scrutiny of how sports historically handled, discussed, and often disguised brain injuries embedded under a cloud of masculinity.

As this book has argued, CTE became a mediated event led by a desire to uncover scientific findings in real time to challenge a global sports industry. In this process, media played a significant role in positioning CTE as a football problem more so than as a concern of repeated blows to the head. Scientific journal articles often referenced media as a cause for public concern and a source of misconception about CTE by reporting on isolated cases through sensationalized stories of toxic deaths, including murder and suicide. The rapid rise in the sheer number of media stories included in this book indicated that media jumped on a popularizing story about the risk of playing football. A symbiotic relationship formed between media and science along the way to the NFL's public acknowledgement and beyond.

A brief survey of the library database at the University of South Florida revealed a parallel rise in academic journal publications of CTE. A search of "chronic traumatic encephalopathy" was conducted across three-year cycles to identify CTE either in an article's title or abstract, which is a short summary of an article's key findings. This is akin to the headline-to-lead relationship in journalism. From 2007 to 2009, only five articles were listed as academic journal publications with CTE in the title or abstract. Between 2010 and 2012, 103 articles mentioned CTE in the abstract, with 38 including it in the title. From 2013 to 2015, academic journals mentioned CTE in 422 abstracts and 86 titles. Finally, between 2016 and 2018, 603 journal publications included CTE in the abstract with 129 in the title.

This simple, yet provocative, finding offers insight into the relationship between science and media in perpetuating CTE as a public health issue of significant concern. It also explains how CTE resulted in an availability cascade of information over data, or as Barr (2013) explained, "a social phenomenon" (p. 271) focused on a sports league cover-up through science and in conflict with science, subsequently played out through media events. Various social forces meet at the intersection of availability cascades that can compound a given phenomenon. In this case, CTE offered a cascade of information about an unknown disease that was circulated and manipulated by powerful organizations and rose to a level of public discourse that, at times, would supersede findings through biased narratives focused on the immediate and drastic effects of storytelling (Kuran & Sunstein, 1999).

Despite concerns that created an availability cascade, the NFL eventually—albeit slowly—moved away from a completely defensive stance of denial to the funding of CTE research, possibly caused by the change in public perception surrounding the safety of the most popular sport. In 2012, the NFL announced a $30-million "unrestricted gift" to the National Institutes of Health (NIH) to study brain injuries. The NFL's press release recognized the league as a "founding donor" for the newly formed NIH Sports and Health Research Program. The donation was the largest philanthropic gift in NFL history ("NFL donates," 2012). In 2013, the NIH announced that it "launched a major effort to define the neuropathological characteristics of CTE" (McKee et al., 2016, p. 77). However, this partnership did not last long.

On July 28, 2017, ESPN reported that the NIH was leaving $16 million of the $30 million donation unspent as "a measure of the mistrust" (Fainaru-Wada & Fainaru, 2017a, para. 3) between the NIH and the NFL. This distrust stemmed from "a bitter dispute" (para. 2) when the NFL backed out of funding for a 2015 study led by Robert Stern, who is part of the CTE Center and a perceived NFL critic. The partnership ended three days after the published study that 99 percent of 111 NFL brains were diagnosed with CTE, of which Stern was listed as one of the article's 27 authors along with Cantu, McKee, and Nowinski (Mez, 2017). In an interview for the show *All Things Considered* on National Public Radio, McKee said, "we know this (CTE) is a problem in football" (Goldman, 2017, para. 14) and she added skepticism of any future NFL-funded research studies because the league was interested only in funding research that they could approve. Specific to the availability cascade of CTE, McKee noted that brains were donated because family members were concerned about seeing reported symptoms of CTE, which produced a skewed population. Despite these biased samples, McKee added that millions of dollars were needed to fund longitudinal studies of CTE. However, those funding opportunities were not guaranteed because "there's so much discussion of this disease *not* existing that funding agencies are reluctant to consider this a real neuro-degenerative disease" (Goldman, 2017, para. 24). This concern of an unknown, and possibly unverified, disease stems from a long-standing, sometimes contentious, relationship between scientists and journalists (Ban et al., 2016; Kuhn et al., 2017).

The battle between scientifically verifiable, unbiased data, how media reports and interprets these findings, and the NFL's response remains at the center of the concern raised by McKee and countless other published authors. The credibility and reliability of CTE research and its effect on the NFL's public perception, long-term viability, and, in a larger context, safety to prevent brain injuries are at the nexus of the data debate (Finkel

& Bienick, 2018). Clearly a link exists between football (and other contact sports) and CTE, which gives credence to the need to determine what—if any—measures can be taken to battle against CTE development in future brains. However, how data are gathered and used in the future can have a social impact on sports participation and the study of brain trauma.

Thus, CTE provided a phenomenon to position media, science, and the NFL in the same predicaments of the two global epidemics outlined in chapter 2. Media is in a unique position to respond to the need for more reliable information regarding CTE. When coupled with a cultural force as strong as professional sports led by the NFL, the ability for individuals to make uninformed assumptions increases. Therefore, it is the duty that media should act as an important public service in restraining from sensationalistic reporting that can further foster uninformed responses to the issue of CTE (Reardon & Richardson, 1991).

PARADOXICAL PARALLELS TO HIV/AIDS AND BIG TOBACCO

As noted throughout this book, media framing of CTE offered several parallels to the case studies of HIV/AIDS and Big Tobacco. First, HIV/AIDS was a prime example of a cascade of information to the public (via media, science, and governmental oversight) that fueled fear of an epidemic that would ravage the United States. It was not until there was a threat to American ideology of masculinity that fear was positioned as the greatest threat from this disease. In the context of AIDS, heterosexuality was championed while homosexuality was condemned, further solidifying sexuality via a heteronormative, masculine lens. Reporting in the 1980s about this global epidemic infecting American soil turned to idealistic stories to position individuals as faces of this disease to personalize it and make it more tangible, and thus, real for the public. Once the number of deaths started to decline and public fear began to subside, it was only in isolated cases that it returned to media spotlight.

CTE has followed a similar narrative arc that appears to have reached its climax and is working toward resolution. Additionally, it is important to note that in the context of HIV/AIDS, by 1994, 70 percent of media stories mentioning AIDS were reporting on something else altogether. As time progressed, AIDS stories became shorter and more focused on celebrities (Brodie et al., 2004). The findings of this book parallel this progression in the context of CTE as more and more stories mentioning CTE emphasize an athlete rather than educating the public on the health issue.

In the context of Big Tobacco, many of the images shared via tobacco advertising, and perpetuated by other forms of mass media, relied upon rugged, independent, and strong images of masculinity to encourage consumers to become addicted to the product. The strongest parallel between Big Tobacco/cancer and NFL/CTE is twofold. First, each global corporation used skewed scientific findings led by medically funded individuals tasked with ensuring long-term opportunities for denial. The parallel between the TIRC and MTBI Committee is eerily similar down to the public relations strategies and personnel utilized by both corporate giants. Second, the strategic approach to rebuild a brand was through notions of corporate social responsibility. For Big Tobacco, it was warning labels on packaging, removal of images that promoted benefits of smoking, and funding research that offered a first step of goodwill after generating billions through spreading cancer. Ultimately, it was through congressional oversight and valid science that Big Tobacco's propaganda was undone. The NFL is in a similar spot and still navigating its murky plan as evident in its handling of the NIH funding.

As was the case with HIV/AIDS, it is possible that media were speculative regarding their coverage of CTE, focusing on attractive headlines rather than delving into the scientific evidence of this budding environmental health risk (Asken & Bauer, 2018). Rather than educate the public about CTE, its definition, its risks, and its long-term effects, media have emphasized the relationship between CTE and the NFL by positioning them as oppositional forces instead of taking the time to learn about the health condition. Much like the coverage of AIDS, it is important to address the frames and subsequent agendas being dictated by media regarding CTE. Many agendas seen in the AIDS case study (e.g., emphasis on isolated cases, media, policy, science, industries) (Rogers et al., 1991) were repeated in the CTE era (Daugherty & Sarmiento, 2018; Randolph, 2018; Solomon, 2018).

The scientific outcomes for HIV/AIDS versus Big Tobacco have largely gone in two different directions. HIV/AIDS research has progressed to a level where an individual can live with HIV and better manage the progression of the virus if provided proper care and treatment. Media portrayals of HIV/AIDS have become somewhat normalized and thus, have decreased—yet when portrayed (e.g., in pop culture), stigma and stereotypes remain (Johnson, 2013). In the case of tobacco use, the link between smoking and cancer is much more direct, resulting in a more linear cause and effect. However, media remain connected to tobacco through its newest iteration with e-cigarettes, which is a growth area for advertising revenue that "can make smoking more acceptable in public again" (Huerta, Walker, Mullen, Johnson, & Ford, 2017, p. 345).

In the case of CTE, science is arguably still in its discovery phase, meaning that much is still not known about its progression and subsequent effects. However, efforts have been made to quantify potential inherent risks between football and CTE as a public health concern despite noted limitations regarding sampling bias (Finkel & Bienick, 2018). This book found that media framing of CTE paralleled that of HIV/AIDS and Big Tobacco in many ways. Particularly, our findings highlight the ways in which the coverage of CTE mimics the progression of HIV/AIDS coverage, where media are currently engaging in the third phase of "crisis management"—which is ironic, considering CTE research is still considered in relative infancy. Here, the NFL continues its attempts at controlling the CTE narrative as science continues to learn more about the diagnosis and its effects. This phase also marks the media's focus on individualized stories associated with CTE (e.g., professional athlete deaths) and offers less information on the scientific findings being unveiled with the progression of time.

Media, by and large because of Congress, have compared the NFL to Big Tobacco, specifically because of the overlap between the two entities in terms of their shared use of lawyers, lobbyists, and public relations playbooks (Fainaru-Wade & Fainaru, 2013; Paolini, 2019; Schwarz, Bogdanich, & Williams, 2016). The entity of Big Tobacco influenced media's subsequent coverage of its public relations crisis, perhaps showing why smoking is the best comparison case with CTE and the NFL. The NFL serves as a close relative of Big Tobacco when considering how the organization has directly influenced the money behind CTE, public questioning of its legitimacy, and the policies surrounding it. However, the NFL faced a twenty-first-century challenge of not being able to deny CTE fast enough, as science continued to move past the organization's statement emphasizing doubt and toward further understanding of the health issue and the risks it poses.

It can be argued that in the case of the NFL and CTE, hegemonic masculinity has played a significant role in why it took so long for the league, media, and public to admit that brain injuries at the professional level are an issue. In a sport that celebrates aggressiveness and toughness, it stands to reason that a brain diagnosis as serious as CTE threatens that very culture. Miller (2014) described the NFL as "a domestically powerful oxymoron of hypermasculinist managerial domination and labor aristocracy" (p. 104). This may help explain media's fascination with constructing CTE as an American football issue that received global coverage. The league found itself at a public relations crossroads where it could no longer drive a self-serving positive media representation because the league was trapped in a spin cycle of constant negative messaging that directly linked the NFL with CTE. To position itself as a hero for acknowledging the problem, the NFL turned to a willingness to work with science rather than against it, at least until it disagreed with the findings or the process. However, it cannot be ignored that the NFL's initial responses defined an era of skepticism and ignorance as Big Tobacco once did (Benson, 2017). In this vein, it becomes even more important that research address how media contextualize the issue of CTE for the public. As Furness (2016) described in examining *League of Denial* as an example of the power of media, the film

> does important work in terms of critiquing both the NFL's institutional and representational practices by advancing a sophisticated, conjunctural analysis that effectively contextualizes the "concussion crisis" with a matrix of economic, historical, cultural and political forces that are rarely part of public debate about professional sport in the United States. (p. 50)

The authors of this book hope it provides similar context to understand CTE within all the social forces at play and can offer a reason for future research to investigate the effects of how media inform audiences about CTE and traumatic brain injuries.

CHALLENGING THE NFL

What is arguably lost in all the mediated and scientific interest in CTE is that it is considered the only preventable form of dementia and is only an environmental hazard (Boston University, 2009; "Often misdiagnosed," 2011). Rarely is this ever mentioned in media or scientific reports. This is not surprising, although disappointing, because to implement a preventative approach would be to eliminate football and other contact sports. This ideological flip is difficult to comprehend for two reasons. First, to eliminate football would mean to release a stranglehold of contact sport, with football as the lynchpin, embedded in American masculine identity and American culture overall. Second, the elimination of football is not likely to happen anytime soon because the industry generates too much revenue, and by extension, financial grants for scientific research to continue.

The concept of America without football is as ideologically opposed as America without democracy. Instead, the discussion around CTE focuses on its cause (e.g., football) and emphasizes that there are no preventative interventions (Montenigro, Bernick, & Cantu, 2015)—other than elimination. Ventresca (2018) explained that by "defining CTE exclusively as a disease, moreover, inevitably invokes notions of a 'cure'" (p. 15). Therefore, while this book focuses on the mediated construction of CTE and how it was framed as a football epidemic, a possible rising concern—and future research opportunity—is how CTE entertains thoughts of another American ideological phenomena of medicalization over prevention.

Multiple state legislators have proposed laws to prohibit tackling before a player becomes a teenager. Medical experts have suggested to not allow children to play tackle football until age 18 or at least refrain from tackling before age twelve (Alosco et al., 2017). With new information released each year, the onus shifts to parents to decide if their children should play tackle football, which has witnessed a substantial decline in youth participation "largely attributed to fears over CTE from concussions" (Lawrence, 2018, p. 126). However, Lawrence follows that declaration with a thought from Robert Stern that concussion is the wrong topic to focus attention. Stern said, "It's concussion this, concussion that. . . . With the focus on concussions, it takes everyone in a different direction from what the real problem is" (p. 126), which Stern said is in the subconcussive impacts that likely occur somewhere on the field during every play. Again, debate of use of concussion and subconcussive hits offers a contested space for scientists to further debate and perpetuate CTE as a disease that needs a cure.

The scientific research community leading the charge against brain injuries in sport appears willing to challenge the NFL, but arguments are made that funding from the league is paramount to understanding the root cause of the problem. What is not mentioned often in media reports is that several of these scientists work with the NFL or receive research money from them. This red flag, hopefully at least tamped down by the MTBI Committee debacle, still offers a specter of doubt when these individuals publish research findings. Beyond the individual researcher is where and how governmental agencies should work with the NFL. For example, Bachynski and Goldberg (2018) raised concern of an NFL partnership between USA Football and the CDC to promote skewed messaging. As the authors asserted, "the NFL's private agenda has influenced how the CDC frames the risks of sports-related brain trauma to the public" (p. 180). Relationships between government agencies and the NFL do not promise a conflict of interest but can raise a concern when—or if—long-term initiatives could influence public trust in reliability or validity of scientific findings.

A few questions are important to consider at this intersection of corporate giants and public institutions. What should the public make of these multibillion-dollar companies and organizations working in conjunction with one another? Where does the line blur between oversight and capitalistic opportunity? Where is media in all of this as the public watchdogs? Why do so few of these organizations explain that CTE is preventable, instead of consistently describing it as a public health concern or crisis? The answer is money. The political economy of American football, namely the NFL, is often at the heart of many of the issues addressed in this book.

Moving beyond the debate over age restrictions for playing tackle football and where money is distributed, a counterargument is often made for the physical benefits of playing sports, albeit contact or other. This argument is grounded in research that has identified poor diet and physical inactivity as the second-leading cause of death in the United States, and it has steadily risen to nearly surpass tobacco as the long-standing leading cause of death (McGinnis & Foege, 1993; Mokdad, Marks, Stroup, & Gerberding, 2004). These facts can be smoke-screened by stories that reach levels of availability cascade to shift focus away from discussions centered around preventable causes of death to sensationalized, media-driven narratives of concern (Kuran & Sunstein, 1999).

FUTURE RESEARCH

This book concludes with the idea that CTE has reached its mediated peak with the NFL and will begin to witness a decline in overall attention focused on football that will further shift to stories of individual demise. Media will continue to unpack the NFL for all its complexity as the last bastion of American masculinity, but CTE will become a subset, not a focal point. Jenkins (2014) provided a parallel to the coal industry to outline the challenge ahead for the NFL and its potential labor pool.

> The NFL has become a public health issue, and that's not an overstatement. Here's why: The league is spending $45 million to sponsor tackle football for children. The league encourages small boys to participate in an activity that beats their heads to pulp and persuades parents that such a thing is okay in order to keep the participation pipeline going. (p. D1)

With Miller's admission of a link between football and CTE, the public received its first hint of NFL guilt. In response, the NFL started targeting youth football participants through "media intensive" (Montez de Oca, Meyer, & Scholes, 2016, p. 4) marketing strategies to sell the benefits of participation and teamwork in a safe environment fostered by the now socially responsible NFL corporation aimed at creating long-term fans. Theoretically, responsibility shifts to those parents and children moving forward to decide if football is worth the risk (Daugherty & Sarmiento, 2018), and the media messages provided by the NFL offer an insightful area of future research.

Public understanding of CTE is a prominent area for future research. Given the dearth of information now available, surveys of players, parents, and coaches offer a first glimpse into the impact of mediated information. Additionally, media campaigns should be created to educate the public about the risks of brain injuries in all sports—not just football—and to help people recognize that the only true prevention of brain injuries is to avoid physical contact. Regarding scientific research, better understanding of all risks, including domestic violence and military members, are necessary to truly paint a public image of CTE. Finally, a better marriage between media presentation of scientific findings is paramount to ensure that the public understands that anyone can be considered at-risk for CTE.

The news stories included in this book offer a potential shift toward the NHL, based on mounting research of CTE diagnoses in hockey players linked to fighting and resulting brain disease. Additionally, the NHL is following the playbook of Big Tobacco and the NFL, as commissioner Gary Bettman continues to deny a link between hockey and CTE. Apparently, it is impossible for multibillion-dollar sport organizations to learn from each other. Instead, hockey is positioned for the next bout with media representation of CTE as a public health epidemic.

Regarding the NFL, the reduction of CTE as a media event is underway. As evident by the decrease in news stories from 2016 to 2017 and again in 2018, this rise and fall of CTE offered an example of what Schudson (1986) described as news events gaining traction through stories "that persist and take different turns over days or weeks or longer" (p. 89). That was CTE until the NFL admitted a link, which posited 2016 as an end of the "binary position" (p. 99) for the CTE narrative as an availability cascade that started in 2005 and will forever be connected to the NFL. Therefore, extensive media studies can begin to contextualize the complex relationship between CTE and the NFL.

FINAL THOUGHT

The penultimate example of CTE, its effect, and ultimate outcome lies in the life and death story of Aaron Hernandez. After signing a $40 million contract before the 2012 season, Hernandez played fourteen games that season for the New England Patriots. On June 17, 2013, Hernandez murdered Odin Lloyd. Nine days later, Hernandez was arrested and charged. On April 26, 2015, Hernandez was convicted of murder and sentenced to life in prison. Less than two years later, on April 19, 2017, Hernandez was found dead in his prison cell after he hanged himself with a bed sheet.

Five months later, on September 21, 2017, McKee announced Hernandez was diagnosed with Stage 3 (of 4) CTE. Just twenty-seven years old at the time of his death, Hernandez had "the first case we've ever seen of that kind of damage in such a young individual" (Barlow, 2017, para. 4). Media continued to report on each of these steps in the Hernandez case, but because of the diagnosis, a few outlets raised the question of whether CTE (and thus, the NFL) could be a defense for murder (Nierenberg, 2017). While this might sound outlandish, it is the point where CTE arrived in media discourse. The cause, side effects, symptoms, and potential long-term effects are already widely available. Thus, Hernandez served as the ultimate case with an awful outcome. Regardless of public perception of Hernandez, where does the media go from here?

Couple the Hernandez findings with stated claims by multiple high school football players—who channeled their inner Jamal Adams—that they were willing to die for football, and regardless of mounting knowledge of long-term brain disease, football remains a significant draw for labor, and, by extension, fans willing to watch the carnage unfold at all levels. Instead of the future labor pool thinking critically about the issue of brain injury in football, many of the elite players—though with some stated opposition—appear to not focus on scientific findings or risk. Instead, they are driven by the hegemonic masculine ideals that have such a firm grasp on the ideology of football and all its mediated splendor that players are willing to risk life in pursuit of a professional dream that is nearly unattainable for the general population. That is something difficult to wrap one's mind around.

References

2012 National Film Registry picks in a league of their own. (2012, December 19). Retrieved December 22, 2017, from https://www.loc.gov/item/prn-12-226/cinematic-firsts-enshrined-in-2012-film-registry/2012-12-19/

A man's game. (1959, November 30). *Time, 74*(22), 58-65.

Adler, R. H., & Herring, S. A. (2011, October). Changing the culture of concussion: Education meets legislation. *Physical Medicine & Rehabilitation, 3*(Suppl. 2), 2468-470.

Adubato, B. (2016). The promise of violence: Televised, professional football games and domestic violence. *Journal of Sport and Social Issues, 40*(1), 22-37.

Ahmed, O. H., & Hall, E. E. (2017). "It was only a mild concussion": Exploring the description of sports concussions in online news articles. *Physical Therapy in Sport, 23*, 7-13.

Albano, Jr., A. W., Adler, R. H., Herring, S. A., & Asif, I. M. (2016). The legal landscape of concussion: Implications for sports medicine providers. *Sports Health, 8*(5), 465-468.

Albicini, M., & McKinlay, A. (2018). A review of sideline assessment measures for identifying sports-related concussions. *Journal of Concussion, 2*, 1-11. https://doi.org/10.1177%2F2059700218784826

Alley, Jr., R. H. (1964, May 4). Head and neck injuries in high school football. *Journal of the American Medical Association, 188*(5), 418-422.

Alosco, M. L., Healy, R. C., & Stern, R. A. (2019). Chronic traumatic encephalopathy and the long-term consequences of repetitive head impacts in sports. In P. A. Arnett (Ed.), *Neuropsychology of sports-related concussion* (pp. 151-182). Washington, D.C.: American Psychological Association.

Alosco, M. L., Kasimis, A. B., Stamm, J. M., Chua, A. S., Baugh, C. M., Daneshvar, D. H.... Stern, R. A. (2017). Age of first exposure to American football and long-term neuropsychiatric and cognitive outcomes. *Translational Psychiatry, 7*, e1236. doi: 10:1038/tp.2017.197

American Academy of Neurology. (2000, May 5). Concussions may spell later trouble for football players. *Science Daily*. Retrieved October 27, 2017, from https://www.sciencedaily.com/releases/2000/05/000505064356.htm

Andelman, D. A. (1994). Big tobacco = big money = big headaches. *Management Review, 83*(10), 48-52.

Anderson, E., & Kian, E. M. (2012). Examining media contestations of masculinity and head trauma in the National Football League. *Men and Masculinities, 15*(2), 152-173.

Andrew, B. C. (2007). Media-generated shortcuts: Do newspaper headlines present another roadblock for low-information rationality? *The International Journal of Press/Politics, 12*(2), 24-43.

Andsager, J. L., & Powers, A. (1999). Social or economic concerns: How news and women's magazines framed breast cancer in the 1990s. *Journalism and Mass Communication Quarterly, 76*, 531-550.

Andsager, J. L., & Powers, A. (2001). Framing women's health with a sense-making approach: Magazine coverage of breast cancer and implants. *Health Communication, 13*, 163-185.

Anshel, M. (2016). *In praise of failure: The value of overcoming mistakes in sports and in life.* Lanham, MD: Rowman & Littlefield.

Anzidei, M. (2018, June 14). Girls are more likely to get concussion in sports, especially soccer, than boys. Retrieved July 31, 2018, from https://www.northjersey.com/story/

sports/high-school/2018/07/14/girls-more-likely-get-concussions-sports-than-boys/764633002/

Arain, M., Haque, M., Johal, L., Mathur, P., Nel, W., Rais, ... Sharma, S. (2013). Maturation of the adolescent brain. *Neuropsychiatric Disease and Treatment, 9*, 449-461.

Armour, N. (2016, March 16). NFL's acknowledgement overdue; CTE's connection to football long had been clear. *USA Today*, p. 3C.

Arthur, P., & Cutler, J. (1995). On the rebound: *Hoop Dreams* and its discontents. *Cinéaste, 21*(3), 22-24.

Arthur, R. (2016, February 29). The shrinking shelf life of NFL players. *The Wall Street Journal*. Retrieved November 13, 2017, from https://www.wsj.com/articles/the-shrinking-shelf-life-of-nfl-players-1456694959

Aschwanden, C. (2016). Women get sports concussions at higher rates than men. *FiveThirtyEight.com*. Retrieved July 13, 2018, from https://fivethirtyeight.com/features/women-get-sports-concussions-at-higher-rates-than-men/

Asken, B. M., & Bauer, R. M. (2018, September). Chronic traumatic encephalopathy: The horse is still chasing the cart. *Journal of Orthopaedic & Sports Physical Therapy, 48*(9), 672-675.

Asken, B. M., Sullan, M. J., DeKosky, S. T., Jaffee, M. S., & Bauer, R. M. (2017). Research gaps and controversies in chronic traumatic encephalopathy: A review. *JAMA Neurology, 74*(10), 1255-1262.

Asplund, C. A., & Best, T. M. (2015, August). Brain damage in American football: Inevitable consequence or avoidable risk? *British Journal of Sports Medicine, 49*(15), 1015-1016.

Axelrod, M. (2001). Popular Culture and the Rituals of American Football. *CLCWeb: Comparative Literature and Culture, 3(1)*, 1-8. Retrieved from http://docs.lib.purdue.edu/clcweb/vol3/iss1/

Bachman, J. (2017). *The New York Times* and *Washington Post*: Misleading the public about US drone strikes. *Journalism Studies, 18*(4), 470-494.

Bachynski, K. E., & Goldberg, D. S. (2018). Time out: NFL conflicts of interest with public health efforts to prevent TBI. *Injury Prevention, 24*(3), 180-184.

Ball, M. A. (2000). Political language and the search for an honorable peace: Presidents Kennedy and Johnson, their advisers, and Vietnam decision making. In C. de Landtsheer & O. Feldman (Eds.), *Beyond public speech and symbols: Explorations in the rhetoric of politicians and the media* (pp. 35-51). Westport, CT: Praeger Publishers.

Ban, V. S., Madden, C. J., Bailes, J. E., Batjer, H. H., & Lonser, R. R. (2016, April). The science and questions surrounding chronic traumatic encephalopathy. *Neurosurgical Focus, 40*(4), E15.

Bardhan, N. (2001). Transnational AIDS-HIV news narratives: A critical exploration of overarching frames. *Mass Communication and Society, 4*, 283-309.

Barlow, R. (2017, November 10). Aaron Hernandez's CTE worst seen by BU experts in a young person. Retrieved December 15, 2017, from http://www.bu.edu/research/articles/aaron-hernandez-cte-worst-seen-in-young-person/

Barnhurst, K. G. (2014). The problem of realist events in American journalism. *Media and Communication, 2*(2), 84-95.

Barone, E. (2017, August). The astronomical cost of kids' sports. *Time*. Retrieved July 13, 2018, from http://time.com/4913284/kids-sports-cost/

Barr, W. B. (2013, December). An evidence based approach to sports concussion: Confronting the availability cascade. *Neuropsychology Review, 23*(4), 271-272.

Bates, T. R. (1975). Gramsci and the theory of hegemony. *Journal of the History of Ideas, 36*(2), 351-366.

Baugh, C. M., Robbins, C. A., Stern, R. A., & McKee, A. C. (2014). Current understanding of chronic traumatic encephalopathy. *Current Treatment Options in Neurology, 16*(306), 1-13.

Beissel, A. S., Giardina, M., & Newman, J. I. (2014). Men of steel: Social class, masculinity, and cultural citizenship in post-industrial Pittsburgh. *Sports in Society, 17*(7), 953-976.

Bell, A. (1991). *The language of news media*. Oxford: Blackwell.

Bell, T. R., & Coche, R. (2018). High power kick: Content analysis of the 2015 USWNT World Cup victory on American front pages. *Communication & Sport*, *6*(6), 745-761.

Bell, T. R., Morales, A. W., & Robb, J. (2017). Communities of practice, media dependency, and surveillance: A virtual search for supremacy in fantasy football. *Reconstruction: Studies in Contemporary Culture*, *17*(1). http://reconstruction.digitalodu.com/issues/contents_171/171_bell_morales_robb/

Bell, T. R., & Sanderson, J. (2016). A hit on American football: A case study of bottom-up framing through op-ed readers' comments. *International Journal of Sport Communication*, *9*(4), 499-518.

Belson, K. (2015, December 17). Ex-player's family says film smears him. *The New York Times*, p. 12B.

Belson, K. (2016, September 27). Researchers make progress toward identifying C.T.E. in the living. *The New York Times*. Retrieved from http://www.nytimes.com/2016/09/27/sports/football/cte-concussions-diagnose-in-living.html

Belson, K., & Schwarz, A. (2016, March 15). NFL shifts on concussions, and game may never be the same. *The New York Times*. Retrieved from https://www.nytimes.com/2016/03/16/sports/nfl-concussions-cte-football-jeff-miller.html

Benson, P. (2017). Big football: Corporate social responsibility and the culture and color of injury in America's most popular sport. *Journal of Sport and Social Issues*, *41*(4), 307-334.

Benton, D. (2017, May 22). Ben Roethlisberger urges NFL players to self-report concussions. *Larry Brown Sports*. Retrieved July 14, 2018, from http://larrybrownsports.com/football/ben-roethlisberger-urges-nfl-players-self-report-concussions/371112

Bernstein, A. L. (2012). Into the red zone: How the National Football League's quest to curb concussions and concussion-related injuries could affect players' legal recovery. *Seton Hall Journal of Sports and Entertainment Law*, *22*(2), 271-309.

Billings, A. C., Angelini, J. R., MacArthur, P. J., Bissell, K., & Smith, L. R. (2014). (Re)calling London: The gender frame agenda within NBC's primetime broadcast of the 2012 Olympiad. *Journalism & Mass Communication Quarterly*, *91*(1), 38-58.

Binney, Z. O., & Bachynski, K. E. (2019). Estimating the prevalence at death of CTE neuropathology among professional football players. *Neurology*, *92*, 1-3. doi: 10.1212/WNL.0000000000006699.

Birkner, T. (2016). Journalism 1914: The birth of modern journalism in Germany a century ago. *Journalism History*, *42*(3), 153-163.

Biswas, J. (2014). Debunking the myths: Oncological misconceptions. *Indian Journal of Medical Research*, *139*, 185-187.

Blakey, S. M., Wagner, H. R., Naylor, J., Brancu, M., Lane, I., Sallee, M., ... Elbogen, E. B. (2018). Chronic pain, TBI, and PTSD in military veterans: A link to suicidal ideation and violent impulses? *The Journal of Pain*, *19*(7), 797-806.

Bodenner, C. (2016, October). How bad are head injuries in soccer? *The Atlantic*. Retrieved from https://www.theatlantic.com/notes/2016/10/how-bad-are-head-injuries-in-soccer/505166/

Bogage, J. (2017, March 27). Girls' soccer, basketball players have higher concussion rates than male counterparts. *Washington Post*. Retrieved July 31, 2018, from https://www.washingtonpost.com/news/recruiting-insider/wp/2017/03/27/girls-soccer-has-highest-concussion-rate-of-high-school-sports-study-finds/

Boggs, W. (2017). Sport-related concussions more common in high school girls. *Reuters*. Retrieved July 13, 2018, from https://www.reuters.com/article/us-health-adolescents-sports-concussions/sport-related-concussions-more-common-in-high-school-girls-idUSKBN17L28V

Boren, C. (2015a, August 16). James Harrison thinks kids' participation trophies are worthless, sets off debate. *Washington Post*. Retrieved July 14, 2018, from https://www.washingtonpost.com/news/early-lead/wp/2015/08/16/james-harrison-wont-let-his-kids-get-participation-trophies/

Boren, C. (2015b, December 2). Ben Roethlisberger sends a powerful message about the NFL's concussion protocol. *Washington Post*. Retrieved November 20, 2016, from https://www.washingtonpost.com/news/early-lead/wp/2015/12/02/ben-roethlisberger-sent-a-powerful-message-about-the-nfls-concussion-protocol/?utm_term=.19564e045030

Boseley, S. (2006, December 8). Expert revered for painstaking work that proved link between smoking and cancer. *The Guardian*. Retrieved from https://www.theguardian.com/science/2006/dec/08/cancer.uk

Boston University. (2009, January 27). Football and progressive brain damage: Tom McHale of NFL suffered from chronic traumatic encephalopathy when he died in 2008. *Science Daily*. Retrieved July 2, 2018 from https://www.sciencedaily.com/releases/2009/01/090127165938.htm

Bowers, J. M. (2014). Chronic traumatic encephalopathy and the future of football. *InSight: Rivier Academic Journal, 10*(2), 1-8.

Boyce, G., Curran, J., & Wingate, P. (Eds.). (1978). *Newspaper history from the seventeenth century to the present day*. London: Constable.

Brandt, A. M. (2007). *The cigarette century: The rise, fall, and deadly persistence of the product that defined America*. New York, NY: Basic Books.

Brandt, A. M. (2012). Inventing conflicts of interest: A history of tobacco industry tactics. *American Journal of Public Health, 102*(1), 63-71.

Brandt, A. (2018, July). How NFL and NBA contracts differ, and what NFL players can do to change it. *Sports Illustrated*. Retrieved July 14, 2018, from https://www.si.com/nfl/2018/07/10/nfl-nba-player-contracts-salary-cap-kirk-cousins-aaron-rodgers-lebron-james-chris-paul

Brittle, C., & Zint, M. (2003). Do newspapers lead with lead? A content analysis of how lead health risks to children are covered. *Journal of Environmental Health, 65*(10), 17-22.

Brodie, M., Hamel, E., Brady, L. A., Kates, J., & Altman, D. E. (2004). AIDS at 21: Media coverage of the HIV epidemic 1981–2002. *Columbia Journalism Review*, supplement to March/April, 1-8.

Brown, J., & Walsh-Childers, K. (1994). Effects of media on personal and public health. In J. Bryant & D. Zillmann (Eds.), *Media effects: Advances in theory and research* (1st ed., pp. 389-415). Hillsdale, NJ: Lawrence Erlbaum Associates.

Brown, K. A., Murphy, B., & Maxwell, L. C. (2018). Tried in the court of public opinion: Effects of involvement in criminal transgressions on athlete images. *Communication & Sport, 6*(3), 283-307.

Brown, P., & Levinson, S. (1978). Universals in language usage: Politeness phenomena. In E. Goody (Ed.), *Questions and politeness: Strategies in social interaction* (pp. 56-310). Cambridge: Cambridge University Press.

Brownell, K. D., & Warner, K. W. (2009). The perils of ignoring history: Big tobacco played dirty and millions died. How similar is big food? *The Milbank Quarterly, 87*(1), 259-294.

Bruzzi, S. (2006). *New documentary* (2nd ed.). London: Routledge.

Buckley, W. E. (1988). Concussions in college football: A multivariate analysis. *The American Journal of Sports Medicine, 16*(1), 51-56.

Burgess, I., Edwards, A., & Skinner, J. (2003). Football culture in an Australian school setting: The construction of masculine identity. *Sport, Education and Society, 8*(2), 199-212.

Burstyn, V. (1999). *The rites of men: Manhood, politics, and the culture of sport*. Toronto: University of Toronto Press.

Butterworth, M. L. (2014). NFL films and the militarization of professional football. In T. P. Oates & Z. Furness (Eds.), *The NFL: Critical and cultural perspectives* (pp. 205-225). Philadelphia, PA: Temple University Press.

Butterworth, M. L. (Ed.). (2017). *Sport and militarism: Contemporary global perspectives*. Abingdon, Oxon: Routledge.

Cabot, M. A. (2011). Barry Bonds vs. the media. *Journal of Mass Media Ethics, 26*(1), 66-70.

Calderwood, C., Murray, A. D., & Stewart, W. (2016). Turning people into couch potatoes is not the cure for sports concussion. *British Journal of Sports Medicine, 50*, 200-201.

Campbell, D., & Walker, T. M. (2016, March 16). Denial of CTE ends. *Denver Post*, p. 2B.

Campbell, R. (2016, February 7). Roger Goodell's couch analogy doesn't sit well with Dave Duerson family. *Chicago Tribune*. Retrieved July 13, 2018, from http://www.chicagotribune.com/sports/football/bears/ct-dave-duerson-roger-goodell-couch-20160207-story.html

Cantu, R. C. (1986). Guidelines for return to contact sports after a cerebral concussion. *The Physician & Sportsmedicine, 14*(10), 75-83.

Cantu, R. C. (2004). Concussion in professional football: Repeat injuries – part 4 [Comments]. *Neurosurgery, 55*(4), 874.

Cantu, R., & Hyman, M. (2012). *Concussion and our kids*. Boston: Mariner Books.

Cantu, R. C., & Register-Mihalik, J. K. (2011, October). Consideration for return-to-play and retirement decisions after concussion. *Physical Medicine & Rehabilitation, 3*(10, Suppl. 2), S440-S444.

Carey, J. W. (1986). The dark continent of American journalism. In R. K. Manoff & M. Schudson (Eds.), *Reading the news: A pantheon guide to popular culture* (pp. 146-196). New York: Pantheon Books.

Carpenter, L. (2018, July 20). TV ratings down, team revenues up: Have protests really hurt the NFL? *The Guardian*. Retrieved December 13, 2018, from https://www.theguardian.com/sport/2018/jul/20/nfl-anthem-protests-revenue-tv-ratings-attendance

Carragee, K. M., & Roefs, W. (2004). The neglect of power in recent framing research. *Journal of Communication, 54*, 214-233.

Carrigan, T., Connell, B., & Lee, J. (1985). Toward a new sociology of masculinity. *Theory and Society, 14*(5), 551-604.

Carson, A. (2017, June). Concussion, dementia and CTE: Are we getting it very wrong? *Journal of Neurology, Neurosurgery, and Psychiatry, 88*(6), 462-464.

Carter, E. (n.d.). They call it pro football. *Index of Film Essays*. Retrieved December 22, 2017, from https://www.loc.gov/programs/national-film-preservation-board/film-registry/index-of-essays/

Carter, M. J. (2013). The hermeneutics of frames and framing: An examination of the media's construction of reality. *Sage Open, 3*(3), 1-12. https://doi.org/10.1177/2158244013487915

Casson, I. R., Pellman, E. J., & Viano, D. C. (2006, November). Chronic traumatic encephalopathy in a National Football League player [Correspondence]. *Neurosurgery, 59*(5), E1152.

Casson, I. R., Siegel, O., Sham, R., Campbell, E. A., Tarlau, M., & DiDomenico, A. (1984, May 25). Brain damage in modern boxers. *The Journal of the American Medical Association, 251*(20), 2663-2667.

Cech, L. B. (2015, October 21). Unconventional sports keep kids active. *The Baltimore Sun*. Retrieved July 13, 2018, from http://www.baltimoresun.com/features/bs-hs-kids-alternative-sports-20151021-story.html

Chronology of professional football. (2017). *2017 NFL Record & Fact Book*, pp. 357-374. Retrieved November 21, 2017, from https://static.nfl.com/static/content/public/photo/2017/08/22/0ap3000000833458.pdf

Clinch, N. G. (1973). *The Kennedy neurosis: A psychological portrait of an American dynasty*. New York: Grosset and Dunlap.

Cohen, B. C. (1963). *The press and foreign policy*. Princeton, NJ: Princeton University Press.

Cohen, J. (1997). The media's love affair with AIDS research: Hope vs. hype. *Science, 275*(5298), 298.

Cohen, J., & You, J. (2018, June 14). Ending AIDS? These three places show the epidemic is far from over. *Science Magazine*. Retrieved from http://www.sciencemag.org/news/2018/06/ending-aids-these-three-places-show-epidemic-far-over

Cole, C. L., & Denny, H. (1994). Visualizing deviance in post-Reagan America: Magic Johnson, AIDS, and the promiscuous world of professional sport. *Critical Sociology, 20*(3), 123-147.

Combs, B., & Slovic, P. (1979). Newspaper coverage of causes of death. *Journalism Quarterly, 56*, 837-849.

Comstock, R. D., Currie, D. W., & Pierpoint, L. A. (2015, September). An evidence-based discussion of heading the ball and concussions in high school soccer. *JAMA Pediatrics, 169*(9), 830-837.

Concannon, L. G., Kaufman, M. S., & Herring, S. A. (2014, September/October). Counseling athletes on the risk of chronic traumatic encephalopathy. *Sports Health, 6*(5), 396-401.

Concussion research and treatment. (2016, March 14). *C-SPAN*. Retrieved July 13, 2018, from https://www.c-span.org/video/?406450-1/hearing-concussions&start=4829

Condotta, B. (2016, March 21). Sherman on Goodell: "He's just a suit." *The Seattle Times*, p. C6.

Conti, D. (2005, February 17). Private staffers back up Wecht. *Pittsburgh Tribune Review*.

Corsellis, J. A. N., Bruton, C. J., & Freeman-Browne, D. (1973). The aftermath of boxing. *Psychological Medicine, 3*, 270-303.

Cottler, L. B., Abdallah, A. B., Cummings, S. M., Barr, J., Banks, R., & Forchheimer, R. (2011). Injury, pain, and prescription opioid use among former National Football League (NFL) players. *Drug and Alcohol Dependence, 116*(1-3), 188-194.

Covassin, T., Moran, R., & Elbin, R. J. (2016). Sex differences in reported concussion injury rates and time loss from participation: An update of the National Collegiate Athletic Association injury surveillance program from 2004–2005 through 2008–2009. *Journal of Athletic Training, 51*(3), 189-194.

Covassin, T., Savage, J. L., Bretzin, A. C., & Fox, M. E. (2018, October). Sex differences in sport-related concussion long-term outcomes. *International Journal of Psychophysiology, 132*(Part A), 9-13.

Crepeau, R. C. (2017). Concussions and football. *On Sport and Society*, 814. Retrieved July 2, 2018, from http://stars.library.ucf.edu/onsportandsociety/814

Critchley, M. (1949). Punch-drunk syndromes: The chronic traumatic encephalopathy of boxers. In C. Vincent (Ed.), *Neuro-chirurgie; Hommage à Clovis Vincent* (pp. 131-141). Paris: Maloine.

Critchley, M. (1957, February 16). Medical aspects of boxing, particularly from a neurological standpoint. *British Medical Journal, 5015*, 357-362.

Croteau, D., & Hoynes, W. (1997). *Media/society: Industries, images, and audiences*. Thousand Oaks, CA: Pine Forge.

Dahlberg, T. (2017, February 3). Toughness only goes so far in concussion hits. *Associated Press*.

Danesi, M. (2012). *Popular culture: Introductory perspectives*. Lanham, MD: Rowman & Littlefield.

Darrow, C. J., Collins, C. L., Yard, E. E., & Comstock, R. D. (2009, September). Epidemiology of severe injuries among United States high school athletes: 2005–2007. *American Journal of Sports Medicine, 37*(9), 1798-1805.

Davis, A. G., Castellani, R. J., & McCrory, P. (2015, June). Neurodegeneration and sport. *Neurosurgery, 76*(6), 643-656.

Davis, K. C. (1999). White filmmakers and minority subjects: Cinema vérité and the politics of irony in "Hoop Dreams" and "Paris is Burning." *South Atlantic Review, 64*(1), 26-47.

Daughtery, J. & Sarmiento, K. (2018). Chronic traumatic encephalopathy: What do parents of youth athletes know about it? *Brain Injury, 32*(13-14), 1773-1779.

Dearing, J. W., & Rogers, E. M. (1992). AIDS and the media agenda. In T. Edgar, M. A. Fitzpatrick, & V. S. Freimuth (Eds.), *AIDS: A communication perspective* (pp. 173-194). Hillsdale, NJ: Lawrence Erlbaum Associates.

DeKosky, S. T., Ikonomovic, M. D., & Gandy, S. (2010, September 30). Traumatic brain injury—Football, warfare, and long-term effects. *The New England Journal of Medicine, 363*(14), 1293-1296.

DeKosky, S. T., Jaffee, M., & Bauer, R. (2018, February 27). Long-term mortality in NFL professional football players: No significant increase, but questions remain. *Journal of the American Medical Association, 319*(8), 773-775.

Deuze, M. (2005). What is journalism? Professional identity and ideology of journalists reconsidered. *Journalism, 6*(4), 442-464.

Doll, R., & Hill, A. B. (1950). Smoking and carcinoma of the lung: A preliminary report. *British Medical Journal, 2*(4682), 739-748. doi: 10.1136/bmj.2.4682.739

Doll, R., & Hill, A. B. (1952). A study of the aetiology of carcinoma of the lung. *British Medical Journal, 2*(4797), 1271-1286.

Doll, R., & Hill, A. B. (1954). The mortality of doctors in relation to their smoking habits: A preliminary report. *British Medical Journal, 1*(4877), 1451-1455.

Doll, R., & Hill, A. B. (1956). Lung cancer and other causes of death in relation to smoking: A second report on the mortality of British doctors. *British Medical Journal, 2*(5001), 1071-1081.

Donaldson, M. (1993). What is hegemonic masculinity? *Theory and Society, 22*(5), 643-657.

Dor, D. (2003). On newspaper headlines as relevance optimizers. *Journal of Pragmatics, 35*(5), 695-721.

Dorman, J. M. (2000). Contagious diseases in competitive sport: What are the risks? *College Health, 49*(3), 105-109.

Downey, M. (1991, November 8). Earvin leaves NBA, but his smile remains. *Los Angeles Times*, p. C1.

Draper, K. (2015, November 10). U.S. soccer bans headers for players under 11 to resolve concussion lawsuit. *Deadspin.com*. Retrieved July 12, 2018, from https://deadspin.com/u-s-soccer-bans-headers-for-players-under-11-to-resolv-1741635694

Drysdale, T. A. (2013). Helmet-to-helmet contact: Avoiding a lifetime penalty by creating a duty to scan active NFL players for chronic traumatic encephalopathy. *Journal of Legal Medicine, 34*, 425-452.

Dubin, J. (2015, December 26). Dave Duerson's family among those who have a problem with "Concussion." Retrieved June 11, 2018, from https://www.cbssports.com/nfl/news/dave-duersons-family-among-those-who-have-a-problem-with-concussion/

Dudo, A. (2015). Scientists, the media, and the public communication of science. *Sociology Compass, 9*(9), 761-775.

Dulac, G. (1997, July 27). Webster's introduction kept light by snappy Bradshaw. *Pittsburgh Post-Gazette*, D-1.

Dunn, I. F., Dunn, G., & Day, A. L. (2006, October). Neurosurgeons and their contributions to modern-day athletics: Richard C. Schneider memorial lecture. *Neurosurgical Focus, 21*(4), 1-6.

Dutta, M. J., & Boyd, J. (2007). Turning "smoking man" images around: Portrayals of smoking in men's magazines as a blueprint for smoking cessation campaigns. *HealthCommunication, 22*(3), 253-263. doi: 10.1080/10410230701626901

Dworkin, S. L., & Wachs, F. L. (1998). "Disciplining the body": HIV-positive male athletes, media surveillance, and the policing of sexuality. *Sociology of Sport Journal, 15*(1), 1-20.

Early retirement: Players call it quits in prime of careers. (2015, July 30). *USA Today*. Retrieved March 20, 2017, from https://www.usatoday.com/story/sports/nfl/2015/07/30/early-retirement-players-call-it-quits-in-prime-of-careers/30869513.

Edelson, S. (2014, January 20). Player safety will secure Goodell's legacy. *USA Today*, 4C.

Edmundson, M. (2014, August 23). Football is America's war game. *Los Angeles Times*. Retrieved July 14, 2018, from http://www.latimes.com/opinion/op-ed/la-oe-edmundson-americas-and-war-connection-20140824-story.html

Ellenbogen, R. G., Berger, M. S., & Batjer, H. H. (2010). The National Football League and concussion: Leading a culture change in contact sports. *World Neurosurgery*, *74*(6), 560-565.

Emanuel, D. (2017, July 3). Study links concussions to irregular menstrual cycles. *CNN.com*. Retrieved July 13, 2018, from https://www.cnn.com/2017/07/03/health/concussions-irregular-menstruation-study/index.html

Eme, R., Gilbertson, K., & Oehler, S. (2013). Persistent cognitive impairment in a multiply concussed female athlete: Is it chronic traumatic encephalopathy? A case study. *The Practitioner Scholar: Journal of Counseling and Professional Psychology*, *2*(1), 43-51.

Emke, I. (2000). Agents and structures: Journalists and the constraints on AIDS coverage. *Canadian Journal of Communication*, *25*, 325-345.

Enck-Wanzer, S. M. (2009). All's fair in love and sport: Black masculinity and domestic violence in the news. *Communication and Critical/Cultural Studies*, *6*(1), 1-18.

Entman, R. M. (1991). Framing US coverage of international news: Contrasts in narratives of the KAL and Iran Air incidents. *Journal of Communication*, *41*(4), 6-27.

Entman, R. M. (1993). Framing: Towards clarification of a fractured paradigm. *Journal of Communication*, *43*(4), 51-58.

Entman, R. M. (2007). Framing bias: Media in the distribution of power. *Journal of Communication*, *57*(1), 163-173.

Epstein, S. (1996). *Impure science: AIDS, activism, and the politics of knowledge*. Berkeley, CA: University of California Press.

Estimated probability of competing in college football. (n.d.). Retrieved February 1, 2018, from http://www.ncaa.org/about/resources/research/football

Evans, S. (2016). Journalistic norms, cultural values, and coverage of climate change in the Philippines. *Environmental Communication*, *10*(4), 492-507.

Fainaru, S., & Fainaru-Wada, M. (2015, August 20). Why former 49er Chris Borland is the most dangerous man in football. Retrieved December 21, 2018, from http://www.espn.com/nfl/story/_/id/13463272/how-former-san-francisco-49ers-chris-borland-retirement-change-nfl-forever

Fainaru-Wada, M. (2011). Serving the public interest when the public does not want to know. *Journal of Mass Media Ethics*, *26*(1), 74-78.

Fainaru-Wada, M. (2017, March 29). Lawyers, others vie for pieces of NFL concussion settlement. Retrieved November 22, 2017, from http://www.espn.com/espn/otl/story/_/id/19029607/billion-dollar-nfl-concussion-settlement-turns-nasty-lawyers-others-vie-pieces-payouts-players

Fainaru-Wada, M., & Fainaru, S. (2013). *League of denial: The NFL, concussions, and the battle for truth*. New York: Three Rivers Press.

Fainaru-Wada, M., & Fainaru, S. (2015, March 17). SF's Chris Borland quits over safety issues. *ESPN.com*. Retrieved July 14, 2018, from http://www.espn.com/espn/otl/story/_/id/12496480/san-francisco-49ers-linebacker-chris-borland-retires-head-injury-concerns

Fainaru-Wada, M., & Fainaru, S. (2017a, July 28). NFL-NIH research partnership set to end with $16M unspent. Retrieved October 9, 2017, from http://www.espn.com/espn/otl/story/_/id/20175509/nfl-donation-brain-research-falls-apart-nih-appears-set-move-bulk-30-million-donation

Fainaru-Wada, M., & Fainaru, S. (2017b, August 31). NFL retakes control of brain research as touted alliance ends. Retrieved November 22, 2017, from http://www.espn.com/espn/otl/story/_/id/20509977/nfl-takes-control-brain-research-100-million-donation-all-ending-partnerships-entities

Feddermann-Dermont, N., Straumann, D., & Dvořák, J. (2014). Return to play management after concussion in football: Recommendations for team physicians. *Journal of Sports Sciences, 32*(13), 1217-1228.

Felberbaum, M. (2014, January 10). Deal reached on tobacco firm corrective statements. *Washington Post*. Retrieved from https://www.washingtonpost.com/business/economy/deal-reached-on-tobacco-firm-corrective-statements/2014/01/10/bc960eca-7a47-11e3-8963-b4b654bcc9b2_story.html?utm_term=.8484071998e5

Fields, S. K. (2008). *Female gladiators: Gender, law, and contact sport in America*. Urbana, IL: University of Illinois Press.

Fink, J. S. (2015). Female athletes, women's sport, and the sport media commercial complex: Have we really "come a long way, baby"? *Sport Management Review, 18*(3), 331-342.

Finkel, A. M. & Bienick, K. F. (2018). A quantitative risk assessment for chronic traumatic encephalopathy (CTE) in football: How public health science evaluates evidence. *Human and Ecological Risk Assessment: An International Journal*. doi: 10.1080/10807039.2018.1456899

Flanagan, L. (2017, August). How students' brains are in danger on the field. *The Atlantic*. Retrieved from https://www.theatlantic.com/education/archive/2017/08/how-students-brains-are-in-danger-on-the-field/536604/

Fleck, L. (1979). *Genesis and development of a scientific fact*. Chicago, IL: University of Chicago Press.

Fogel, C. (2011). Sporting masculinity on the gridiron: Construction, characteristics and consequences. *Canadian Social Science, 7*(2), 1-14.

Football not only sport concussion risk for teens. (2012, February). *Reuters*. Retrieved July 13, 2018, from https://www.reuters.com/article/us-concussion-teens/football-not-only-sport-concussion-risk-for-teens-idUSTRE81G06420120217

Foote, J. G., Butterworth, M. L., & Sanderson, J. (2017). Adrian Peterson and the "wussification of America": Football and myths of masculinity. *Communication Quarterly, 65*(3), 268-284.

Foreman, C. (2005, September 2). Pathologist: Fayette girl's injuries were not an accident. *Pittsburgh Tribune Review*.

Fortuna, C. (2015). Digital media literacy in a sports, popular culture and literature course. *Journal of Media Literacy Education, 6*(3), 81-89.

Foster, J. B., Leiguarda, R., & Tilley, P. J. B. (1976, May 8). Brain damage in national hunt jockeys. *The Lancet, 307*(7967), 981-983.

Fox, M. (2018, July 31). Heading a soccer ball harms women more than men, study finds. Retrieved July 31, 2018, from https://www.nbcnews.com/health/health-news/heading-soccer-ball-harms-women-more-men-study-finds-n896236.

Friedman, S. (2016). Head games. [Review of the film *Head Games*, 2012]. *Journal of Sport History, 43*(1), 97-99.

Furness, Z. (2016). Reframing concussions, masculinity, and NFL mythology in *League of Denial*. *Popular Communication, 14*(1), 49-57.

Gaetz, M. (2017, May). The multi-factorial origins of chronic traumatic encephalopathy (CTE) symptomology in post-career athletes: The athlete post-career adjustment (AP-CA) model. *Medical Hypotheses, 102*, 130-143.

Game changers: Stats, stories and what communities are doing to protect young athletes. (2013, August). Retrieved April 15, 2016, from https://www.safekids.org/research-report/game-changers-stats-stories-and-what-communities-are-doing-protect-young-athletes.

Gamson, W. A., Croteau, D., Hoynes, W., & Sasson, T. (1992). Media images and the social construction of reality. *Annual Review of Sociology, 18*, 373-393.

Gamson, W. A., & Modigliani, A. (1987). The changing culture of affirmative action. In R. G. Braungart & M. M. Braungart (Eds.), *Research in political sociology: A research annual* (Vol. 3, pp. 137-177). Greenwich, CT: JAI Press.

Gamson, W. A., & Modigliani, A. (1989). Media discourse and public opinion on nuclear power: A constructionist approach. *American Journal of Sociology, 95*(1), 1-37.

Gans, H. J. (1979). *Deciding what's news: A study of CBS Evening News, NBC Nightly News, Newsweek, and Time.* New York: Random House.

Gardetto, D. C. (1997). Hillary Rodham Clinton, symbolic gender politics, and the *New York Times*: January–November 1992. *Political Communication, 14*(2), 225-240.

Gardner, A., Iverson, G. L., & McCrory, P. (2014, January). Chronic traumatic encephalopathy in sport: A systematic review. *British Journal of Sports Medicine, 48*(2), 84-90.

Gardner, E. C. (2015). Head, face, and eye injuries in collegiate women's field hockey. *The American Journal of Sports Medicine, 43*(8), 2027-2034.

Gavett, B. E., Stern, R. A., Cantu, R. C., Nowinski, C. J., & McKee, A. C. (2010). Mild traumatic brain injury: A risk factor for neurodegeneration. *Alzheimer's Research & Therapy, 2*, 18-21.

Gems, G. R. (2000). *For pride, profit, and patriarchy: Football and the incorporation of American cultural values.* Landham, MD: Scarecrow Press.

Gerberich, S. G., Priest, J. D., Boen, J. R., Straub, C. P., & Maxwell, R. E. (1983, December). Concussion incidences and severity in secondary school varsity football players. *American Journal of Public Health, 73*(12), 1370-1375.

Gessel, L. M., Fields, S. K., Collinc, C. L., Dick, R. W., & Comstock, R. D. (2007). Concussions among United States high school and collegiate athletes. *Journal of Athletic Training, 42*(4), 495-503.

Gilbert, F., & Johnson, S. M. (2011). The impact of American tackle football-related concussions in youth athletes. *AJOB Neuroscience, 2*(4), 48-59.

Gitlin, T. (1980). *The whole world is watching: Mass media in the making & unmaking of the new left.* Berkeley, CA: University of California Press.

Glaser, B. G., & Holton, J. (2004). Remodeling grounded theory. *Forum: Qualitative Social Research, 5*(2). Retrieved from http://www.qualitative-research.net/index.php/fqs/article/view/607

Glaser, B. G., & Strauss, A. L. (1967). *The discovery of grounded theory: Strategies for qualitative research.* New York: AldineTransaction.

Global Statistics. (n.d.). Retrieved December 15, 2018, from https://www.hiv.gov/hiv-basics/overview/data-and-trends/global-statistics

Goffman, E. G. (1956). *The presentation of self in everyday life.* Edinburgh: University of Edinburgh Social Sciences Research Centre.

Goffman, E. G. (1974). *Frame analysis: An essay on the organization of experience.* New York: Harper & Row.

Goldberg, D. S. (2013). Mild traumatic brain injury, the national football league, and the manufacture of doubt: An ethical, legal, and historical analysis. *The Journal of Legal Medicine, 34*, 157-191. doi: 10.1080/01947648.2013.800792

Goldman, T. (2017, July 25). Study: CTE found in nearly all donated NFL player brains. Retrieved October 9, 2017, from http://www.npr.org/2017/07/25/539198429/study-cte-found-in-nearly-all-donated-nfl-player-brains

Goldstein, L. E., Fisher, A. M., Tagge, C. A., Zhang, X., Velisek, L., Sullivan, J. A., … McKee, A. C. (2012). Chronic traumatic encephalopathy in blast-exposed military veterans and a blast neurotrauma mouse model. *Science Translational Medicine, 4*(134), 1-16.

Goodell, R. (1987). The role of mass media in scientific controversies. In H. T. Engelhardt, Jr., & A. L. Caplan (Eds.), *Scientific controversies: Case studies in the resolution and closure of disputes in science and technology* (pp. 585-597). New York: Cambridge University Press.

Gordon, A. (2014, January 22). Did football cause 20 deaths in 1905? Re-investigating a serial killer. *Deadspin.* Retrieved January 15, 2016, from https://deadspin.com/did-football-cause-20-deaths-in-1905-re-investigating-1506758181.

Graham, R. F. (2016, March 20). "He's just a suit": Richard Sherman hits out at Roger Goodell over his 'foolish' proposal to eject players when they commit two personal fouls. *The Daily Mail.* Retrieved June 23, 2018, from http://www.dailymail.co.uk/news/article-3501955/He-s-just-suit-NFL-star-Richard-Sherman-hits-against-commissioner-foolish-ejection-proposal-players.html

Granier, J. P., Mcnamee, S., Cifu, D. X., & Goldberg, G. (2011). Leaping too far too soon. *AJOB Neuroscience*, *2*(4), 60-61.

Grasgreen, A. (2013, December 4). It's not just football. Retrieved July 13, 2018, from https://www.insidehighered.com/news/2013/12/04/experts-work-address-concussions-all-sports-not-just-football

Greenwood, J. K. (2005, September 16). Long autopsy results stir controversy. *Pittsburgh Tribune Review*.

Groothuis, D. (2014, October 21). Violence of football is becoming too difficult to justify. *The Denver Post*. Retrieved July 14, 2018, from https://www.denverpost.com/2014/10/21/violence-of-football-is-becoming-too-difficult-to-justify/

Grossberg, L., Wartella, E., Whitney, D. C., & Wise, J. M. (2006). *Mediamaking: Mass media in a popular culture*. Thousand Oaks, CA: Sage.

Gurevitch, M., & Levy, M. R. (Eds.). (1985). *Mass communication review yearbook* (Vol. 5). Beverly Hills, CA: Sage.

Guskiewicz, K. M. (2001, January). Concussion in sport: The grading-system dilemma. *Athletic Therapy Today*, *6*(1), 18-27.

Guskiewicz, K. M., Marshall, S. W., Bailes, J., McCrea, M., Cantu, R. C., Randolph, C., & Jordan, B. D. (2005). Association between recurrent concussion and late-life cognitive impairment in retired professional football players. *Neurosurgery*, *57*(4), 719-726. doi: 10.1227/01.NEU.0000175725.75780.DD

Guskiewicz, K. M., Marshall, S. W., Bailes, J., McCrea, M., Harding, H. P., Matthews, A., … & Cantu, R. (2007). Recurrent concussion and risk of depression in retired professional football players. *Medicine & Science in Sports Exercise*, *39*(6), 903-909. doi: 10.1249/mss.0b013e3180383da5

Guskiewicz, K. M., McCrea, M., Marshall, S. W., Cantu, R. C., Randolph, C., Barr, W., … Kelly, J. P. (2003, November 19). Cumulative effects associated with recurrent concussion in collegiate football players: The NCAA concussion study. *Journal of the American Medical Association*, *290*(10), 2549-2555.

Guskiewicz, K. M., Weaver, N. L., Padua, D. A., & Garrett, Jr., W. E. (2000). Epidemiology of concussion in collegiate and high school football players. *The American Journal of Sports Medicine*, *28*(5), 643-650.

Gusterson, H. (2013). Anthropology in the news? *Anthropology Today*, *29*(6), 11-13.

Guttmann, A. (2006). Civilized mayhem: Origins and early development of American football. *Sport in Society*, *9*(4), 533-541.

Habib, H. (2015, December 22). Andre Waters' loved ones denounce portrayal of him in "Concussion" movie. *Palm Beach Post*. Retrieved June 11, 2018, from https://www.mypalmbeachpost.com/sports/football/andre-waters-loved-ones-denounce-portrayal-him-concussion-movie/d3WEVrHRAtPLhYVQzv83NL/

Halley, J. (2015, June 16). New study shows women's lacrosse as the No. 2 sport for concussions behind only football. *USA Today High School Sports*. Retrieved July 13, 2018, from https://usatodayhss.com/2015/new-study-shows-womens-lacrosse-as-the-no-2-sport-for-concussions-behind-only-football

Hargreaves, J. (1997). Women's boxing and related activities: Introducing images and meanings. *Body and Society*, *3*(4), 33-49.

Harmon, K. G., Drezner, J. A., Gammons, M., Guskiewicz, K. M., Halstead, M., Herring, S. A., … Roberts, W. O. (2013, January). American Medical Society for Sports Medicine position statement: Concussion in sport. *British Journal of Sports Medicine*, *47*(1), 15-26.

Harrison, E. A. (2014, May). The first concussion crisis: Head injury and evidence in early American football. *American Journal of Public Health*, *104*(5), 822-833.

Hart, C. (1998). *Doing a literature review: Releasing the social science research imagination*. London: Sage.

Haskins, J. B. (1966). Headline-and-lead scanning vs. whole-item reading in newspaper content analysis. *Journalism Quarterly*, *43*(2), 333-335.

Hazrati, L., Tartaglia, M. C., Diamandia, P., Davis, K. D., Green, R. E., Wennberg, R., … Tator, C. H. (2013, May). Absence of chronic traumatic encephalopathy in retired football players with multiple concussions and neurological symptomatology. *Frontiers in Human Neuroscience, 7*. Retrieved June 8, 2018, from https://www.frontiersin.org/articles/10.3389/fnhum.2013.00222/full

Heads up. (n.d.). *Center for Disease Control and Prevention*. Retrieved September 5, 2017, from https://www.cdc.gov/headsup/index.html

Healy, M. (2013, August 6). 1.35 million youths a year have serious sports injuries. *USA Today*. Retrieved July 13, 2018, from https://www.usatoday.com/story/news/nation/2013/08/06/injuries-athletes-kids-sports/2612429/

Hears football men. (1905, October 15). *Washington Post*.

Hedges, L. V. (1987). How hard is hard science, how soft is soft science? The empirical cumulativeness of research. *The American Psychologist, 42*(2), 443-455.

Heeter, C., Perlstadt, H., & Greenberg, B. S. (1984, August). *Health incidents, stages of illness and treatment on popular television programs*. Paper presented at the annual convention of the International Communication Association, New Orleans, Louisiana.

Heinemann, A. W., Magasi, S., Hammel, J., Carlozzi, N. E., Garcia, S. F., Hahn, E. A… Jerousek, S. (2015). Environmental factors item development for persons with stroke, traumatic brain injury, and spinal cord injury. *Archives of Physical Medicine and Rehabilitation, 96*, 589-595.

Heiner, J. A. (2008). Concussions in the National Football League: *Jani v. Bert Bell/Pete Rozelle NFL Player Ret. Plan* and a legal analysis of the NFL's 2007 concussion management guidelines. *Seton Hall Journal of Sports and Entertainment Law, 18*(1), 255-296.

Heinze, K. L., & Lu, D. (2017). Shifting responses to institutional change: The National Football League and player concussions. *Journal of Sport Management, 31*(5), 497-513.

Hernández, L. H., & de los Santos Upton, S. (2018). *Challenging reproductive control and gendered violence in the Américas: Intersectionality, power, and struggles for rights*. Lanham, MD: Lexington Books.

Hester, R. D. (2017). Lack of access to mental health services contributing to the high suicide rates among veterans. *International Journal of Mental Health Systems, 11*: 47. doi: 10.1186/s13033-017-0154-2

Higgins, J. W., Naylor, P. J., Berry, T., O'Connor, B., & Mclean, D. (2006). The health buck stops where? Thematic framing of health discourse to understand the context for CVD prevention. *Journal of Health Communication, 11*, 343-358.

Hill, J. W., Darrow, R. W., Thompson, C., & Hoyt, W. T. (1962, February 26). Smoking health and statistics: The story of the tobacco accounts. Lorillard. Bates No. 98721513/1551. Retrieved from https://www.industrydocumentslibrary.ucsf.edu/tobacco/docs/#id=tyfl0060

Hippocrates, C. (1999). Public journalism: The media's intellectual journey. *Media International Australia, Incorporating Culture and Policy, 90*, 65-78.

Hof, P. R., Knabe, R., Bovier, P., & Bouras, C. (1991). Neuropathological observations in a case of autism presenting with self-injury behavior. *Acta Neurpathologica, 82*(4), 321-326.

Hornbeck, K., Walter, K., & Myrvik, M. (2017, July). Should potential risk of chronic traumatic encephalopathy be discussed with young athletes? *AMA Journal of Ethics, 19*(7), 686-692.

Huerta, T. R., Walker, D. M., Mullen, D., Johnson, T. J., & Ford, E. W. (2017). Trends in e-cigarette awareness and perceived harmfulness in the U.S. *American Journal of Preventive Medicine, 52*(3), 339-346.

Hyland, K. (1996). Writing without conviction? Hedging in science research articles. *Applied Linguistics, 17*(4), 433-454.

Ifantidou, E. (2009). Newspaper headlines and relevance: Ad hoc concepts in ad hoc contexts. *Journal of Pragmatics, 41*, 699-720.

"Iron Mike" Mike Webster. (n.d.). Retrieved August 18, 2017, from http://www.profootballhof.com/players/mike-webster/

Iverson, G. L. (2016). Suicide and chronic traumatic encephalopathy. *Journal of Neuropsychiatry and Clinical Neurosciences, 28*(1), 9-16.
Iverson, G. L., Keene, C. D., Perry, G., & Castellani, R. J. (2018). The need to separate chronic traumatic encephalopathy neuropathology from clinical features. *Journal of Alzheimer's Disease, 61*(1), 17-28.
Iyengar, S., & Kinder, D. R. (1987). *News that matters: Television and American opinion.* Chicago: Chicago University Press.
Jadad, A. R., & Enkin, M. W. (2007). *Randomized controlled trials: Questions, answers, and musings* (2nd ed.). Malden, MA: Blackwell Publishing.
Jamal Adams on player safety. (2017, July 31). Retrieved November 13, 2017, from https://www.sny.tv/video/1672122983/jamal-adams-on-player-safety
James, S., & Sheridan, B. (Producers), James, S. (Director). (2012). [Motion Picture]. *Head games: The global concussion crisis.* United States: Variance Films.
Jani v. Bert Bell/Pete Rozelle NFL player retirement plan, 209 Fed. Appx. 305, 40 EBC 2049 (4th Cir. 2006).
Jansen, S. C., & Sabo, D. (1994). The sport/war metaphor: Hegemonic masculinity, the Persian Gulf War, and the new world order. *Sociology of Sport Journal, 11*(1), 1-17.
Jenkins, E. F. (2013). Only the headstrong survive: The tragic course of head injury claims under the Bert Bell/Pete Rozelle NFL player retirement plan. *Syracuse Law Review, 63,* 327-352.
Jenkins, S. (2014, October 2). CTE is NFL's modern version of black lung. *Washington Post,* p. D1.
Jenkins, S. (2016, February 6). On head trauma, Goodell couches neglect in nonsense. *Washington Post,* p. D1.
Jhally, S. (1984). The spectacle of accumulation: Material and cultural factors in the evolution of the sports/media complex. *Critical* Sociology, *12*(3), 41-57.
Jhally, S. (1989). Cultural studies and the sports/media complex. In L. A. Wenner (Ed.), *Media, sports, & society* (pp. 70-93). Newbury Park, CA: Sage.
Joffe, H. (1995). Social representations of AIDS: Towards encompassing issues of power. *Papers on Social Representations, 4*(1), 29-40.
Joffe, H. (1996). Social representation and the AIDS field. *Psychology in Society, 24,* 21-39.
Johnson, C. (2017, April 19). Athletic options for kids who have no interest in traditional team sports. *Washington Post.* Retrieved July 13, 2018, from https://www.washingtonpost.com/news/parenting/wp/2017/04/19/athletic-options-for-kids-who-have-no-interest-in-traditional-team-sports/?utm_term=.9368818d00ae
Johnson, J. (1969). Organic psychosyndromes due to boxing. *The British Journal of Psychiatry, 115*(518), 45-53.
Johnson, M. A. (2013). More than pop culture: Depictions of HIV in the media and the effect on viewer's perception of risk. *Journal of Homosexuality, 60*(8), 1117-1142.
Johnson, V. E. (2016). "Together, We Make Football": The NFL's "feminine" discourses. *Popular Communication, 14*(1), 12-20.
Johnston, J., & Graham, C. (2012). The new, old journalism. *Journalism Studies, 13*(4), 517-533.
Jonsen, A. R., Cooke, M., & Koenig, B. A. (1986). Aids and ethics. *Issues in Science and Technology, 2,* 56-65.
Judge, C. (2017, February 1). Tagliabue exclusive: My 1994 concussions remarks "a mistake." *Talk of Fame Sports Network.* Retrieved November 21, 2017, from http://www.talkoffamenetwork.com/tagliabue-exclusive-1994-concussions-remarks-mistake/
Jung, M. (2013). Framing, agenda setting, and disease phobia of AIDS-related coverage in the South Korean mass media. *The Health Care Manager 32*(1), 52-57.
Kain, D. J. (2009). "It's just a concussion:" The national football league's denial of a causal link between multiple concussions and later-life cognitive decline. *Rutgers Law Journal, 40*(3), 697-736.
Kane, M. (1960, April 24). The end of college boxing. *Sports Illustrated, 7,* 18-19.

Kane, M. J. (1988). Media coverage of the female athlete before, during, and after Title IX: *Sports Illustrated* revisited. *Journal of Sport Management, 2*(2), 87-99.

Kapadia, S. (2016, March 20). Richard Sherman on Roger Goodell's proposal: "He's just a suit." Retrieved June 23, 2018, from http://www.espn.com/nfl/story/_/id/15025641/seattle-seahawks-cb-richard-sherman-rips-roger-goodell-new-rules

Karimipour, N., & Hull, K. (2017). Minimized, not medicalized: Media framing of concussions in the NFL on ESPN.com. *Journal of Sports Media, 12*(2), 45-77.

Katz, B. P., Kudela, M., Harezlak, J., McCrea, M., McAllister, T., & Broglio, S. P. (2018, August). Baseline performance of NCAA athletes on a concussion assessment battery: A report from the CARE consortium. *Sports Medicine, 8*, 1971-1985.

Kearney, M. H. (2017). Challenges of finding and filling a gap in the literature. *Research in Nursing & Health, 40*(5), 393-395.

Keck, K. (2009, June 19). Big tobacco: A history of its decline. *CNN*. Retrieved from http://edition.cnn.com/2009/POLITICS/06/19/tobacco.decline

Keene, C. D., Latimer, C. S., Steele, L. M., & MacDonald, C. L. (2018, February). First confirmed case of chronic traumatic encephalopathy in a professional bull rider. *Acta Neuropathologica, 135*(2), 303-305.

Keith, L. (2010). Foreword. In M. Teitelbaum, *Sports in America, 1980-1989* (2nd ed.) (pp. 4-5). New York: Chelsea House.

Kellett, P. (2002). Football-as-war, coach-as-general: Analogy, metaphor and management implications. *Football Studies, 5*(1), 60-76.

Kemper, K. E. (2009). *College football and American culture in the Cold War era*. Urbana, IL: University of Illinois Press.

Kennedy, E., & Hills, L. (2009). *Sport, media and society*. Oxford: Berg.

Kimmel, M. S., & Messner, M. A. (Eds.). (1992). *Men's lives* (2nd ed.). New York: Macmillan.

King, S., Carey, R. S., Jinnah, N., Millington, R., Phillipson, A., Prouse, C., & Ventresca, M. (2014). When is a drug not a drug? Troubling silences and unsettling painkillers in the National Football League. *Sociology of Sport Journal, 31*(3), 249-266.

Kinnick, K. N., Krugman, D. M., & Cameron, G. T. (1996). Compassion fatigue: Communication and burnout toward social problems. *Journalism and Mass Communication Quarterly, 73*, 687-707.

Kirk, M., Gilmore, J., & Wiser, M. (Producers), Kirk, M. (Director). (2013). *League of denial* [Motion Picture]. United States: Public Broadcasting Service.

Klaidman, S. (1991). *Health in the headlines: The stories behind the stories*. New York, NY: Oxford University Press.

Kline, N. (2003). Popular media and health: Images, effects, and institutions. In T. L. Thompson, A. M. Dorsey, K. I. Miller, & R. Parrott (Eds.), *Handbook of health communication* (pp. 557-581). Mahwah, NJ: Lawrence Erlbaum Associates, Inc.

Knollman-Porter, K., Brown, J., & Flynn, M. (2018). A preliminary examination of concussion knowledge by collegiate athletes and non-athletes. *American Journal of Speech-Language Pathology, 27*, 778-795.

Korngold, C., Farrell, H. M., & Fozdar, M. (2013). The National Football League and chronic traumatic encephalopathy: Legal implications. *The Journal of the American Academy of Psychiatry and the Law, 41*(3), 430-436.

Kovach, B., & Rosenstiel, T. (2007). *The elements of journalism: What newspeople should know and the public should expect*. New York: Three Rivers Press.

Krishnan, S. P., Durrah, T., & Winkler, K. (1997). Coverage of AIDS in popular African American magazines. *Health Communication, 9*, 273-288.

Kroshus, E., Baugh, C. M., Stein, C. J., Austin, S. B., & Calzo, J. P. (2017). Concussion reporting, sex, and conformity to traditional gender norms in young adults. *Journal of Adolescence, 54*, 110-119.

Kroshus, E., Rivara, F. P., Whitlock, K. B., Herring, S. A., & Chrisman, S. P. (2017, November). Disparities in athlete trainer staffing in secondary school sport: Implications for concussion identification. *Clinical Journal of Sport Medicine, 27*(6), 542-547.

Kucera, K. L., Klossner, D., Colgate, B., & Cantu, R. C. (2017). *Annual survey of football injury research, 1931–2016*. Chapel Hill, NC: National Center for Catastrophic Sport Injury Research. Retrieved September 19, 2017, from https://nccsir.unc.edu/files/2013/10/Annual-Football-2016-Fatalities-FINAL.pdf

Kuhn, A. W., Yengo-Kahn, A. M., Kerr, Z. Y., & Zuckerman, S. L. (2017, December). Sports concussion research, chronic traumatic encephalopathy and the media: Repairing the disconnect. *British Journal of Sports Medicine, 51*(24), 1732-1733.

Kuran, T., & Sunstein, C. R. (1999). Availability cascades and risk regulation. *Stanford Law Review, 51*, 683-768.

Kwon, D. (2017, October 2). Concussion recovery is slower in girls, mounting evidence suggests. *Scientific American*. Retrieved July 13, 2018, from https://www.scientificamerican.com/article/concussion-recovery-is-slower-in-girls-mounting-evidence-suggests/

Labra, O. (2015). Social representations of HIV/AIDS in mass media: Some important lessons for caregivers. *International Social Work, 58*(2), 238-248. doi: 10.1177/0020872813497380

Lagerwerf, L., Timmerman, C., & Bosschaert, A. (2016). Incongruity in news headings. *Journalism Practice, 10*(6), 782-804.

Laker, S. R. (2011, October). Epidemiology of concussion and mild traumatic brain injury. *Physical Medicine and Rehabilitation, 3*, S354-S358.

Laskas, J. M. (2009, September 14). Game brain. *GQ*. Retrieved June 11, 2018, from https://www.gq.com/story/nfl-players-brain-dementia-study-memory-concussions

Laskas, J. M. (2015). *Concussion*. New York: Random House.

Lau, E. (2016, June). A head-on collision with the National Football League. *The Lancet Neurology, 15*(7), 669.

Lawrence, A. (2018, July/August). This boy's life. *Men's Health, 33*(6), 122-127, 135.

Leavy, J. (2012, August 17). The woman who would save football. *Grantland.com*. Retrieved June 8, 2018, from http://grantland.com/features/neuropathologist-dr-ann-mckee-accused-killing-football-be-sport-only-hope/

Leech, G. (2014). *The pragmatics of politeness*. Oxford: Oxford University Press.

Lehman, E. J., Hein, M. J., Baron, S. L., & Gersic, C. M. (2012, November 6). Neurodegenerative causes of death among retired National Football League players. *Neurology, 79*(19), 1970-1974.

LePoire, B. (1994). Attraction toward and nonverbal stigmatization of gay males and persons with AIDS: Evidence of symbolic over instrumental attitudinal structures. *Human Communication Research, 21*, 241-279.

Leung, R. (2004, January 26). NFL Films, Inc. *CBS News*. Retrieved December 22, 2017, from https://www.cbsnews.com/news/nfl-films-inc-26-01-2004/

Levin, B., & Bhardwaj, A. (2014). Chronic traumatic encephalopathy: A critical appraisal. *Neurocritical Care, 20*, 334-344.

Lew, H. L., Otis, J. D., Tun, C., Kerns, R. D., Clark, M. E., & Cifu, D. X. (2009). Prevalence of chronic pain, posttraumatic stress disorder, and persistent postconcussive symptoms in OIF/OEF veterans: Polytrauma clinical triad. *Journal of Rehabilitation Research & Development, 46*(6), 697-702.

Lewis, L. A. (Ed.). (1992). *The adoring audience: Fan culture and popular media*. London: Routledge.

Lichtenstein, S., Slovic, P., Fischoff, B., Layman, M., & Combs, B. (1978). Judged frequency of lethal events. *Journal of Experimental Psychology, 4*, 551-577.

Love, S., & Solomon, G. S. (2014). Talking with parents of high school football players about chronic traumatic encephalopathy. *The American Journal of Sports Medicine, 43*(5), 1260-1264.

MacArthur, P. J., Angelini, J. R., Billings, A.C., & Smith, L. R. (2016). The dwindling Winter Olympic divide between male and female athletes: The NBC broadcast network's primetime coverage of the 2014 Sochi Olympic Games. *Sport in Society, 19*(10), 1556-1572.

MacDonald, J., & Myer, G. D. (2017, October). "Don't let kids play football": A killer idea. *British Journal of Sports Medicine, 51*(20), 1448-1449.

Macur, J. (2014, June 25). Setting a new bar on the risks of heading. *New York Times*, B11.

Maese, R. (2014, November 20). Proposed concussion deal draws fire over CTE issue. *Washington Post*, p. D5.

Maese, R. (2016, March 3). Soccer star Brandi Chastain pledges to donate her brain to CTE research for women. *The Washington Post*. Retrieved July 12, 2018, from https://www.washingtonpost.com/sports/dcunited/brandi-chastain-pledges-to-donate-brain-to-concussion-research/2016/03/02/a17affac-e0d3-11e5-8c00-8aa03741dced_story.html?utm_term=.f357815fe7cf

Malec, M. M. (1995). Hoop shots and last dreams. *Journal of Sport & Social Issues, 19*(3), 307-312.

Mandell, N. (2017, August 1). Martellus Bennett had a wise response to rookie who said he would die for football. *USA Today*. Retrieved November 13, 2017, from http://ftw.usatoday.com/2017/08/martellus-bennett-had-a-wise-response-to-rookie-who-said-he-would-die-for-football

Mannix, R., Meehan III, W. P., & Pascual-Leone, A. (2016, August). Sports-related concussions—Media, science and policy. *Nature Reviews Neurology, 12*(8), 486-490.

Manoff, R. K., & Schudson, M. (Eds.). (1986). *Reading the news: A pantheon guide to popular culture*. New York: Pantheon Books.

Markovic, G., Schult., M., & Bartfai, A. (2017). The effect of sampling bias on generalizability in intervention trials after brain injury. *Brain Injury, 31*(1), 9-15.

Maron, B. J. (2015, November). Historical perspectives on sudden deaths in young athletes with evolution over 35 years. *The American Journal of Cardiology, 116*(9), 1461-1468.

Marshall, S. W., Guskiewicz, K. M., Shankar, V., McCrea, M., & Cantu, R. C. (2015). Epidemiology of sports-related concussion in seven US high school and collegiate sports. *Injury Epidemiology, 2*(13). https://doi.org/10.1186/s40621-015-0045-4

Martland, H. S. (1928). Punch drunk. *Journal of the American Medical Association, 91*, 1103-1107.

Marx, G. (2011, November/December). Power of dispassion: Alan Schwarz changed football. *Columbia Journalism Review, 50*(4), 109-112.

Mazerolle, S. M., Raso, S. R., Pagnotta, K. D., Stearns, R. L., & Casa, D. J. (2015). Athletic directors' barriers to hiring athlete trainers in high school. *Journal of Athletic Training, 50*(10), 1059-1068.

McCandless, P. M., Yerger, V. B., & Malone, R. E. (2012). Quid pro quo: Tobacco companies and the black press. *American Journal of Public Health, 102*(4), 739-750.

McChesney, R. W. (1989). Media made sport: A history of sports coverage in the United States. In L. A. Wenner (Ed.), *Media, sports, and society* (pp. 49-69). Newbury Park, CA: Sage.

McClincy, M. P., Lovell, M. R., Pardini, J., Collins, M. W., & Spore, M. K. (2006). Recovery from sports concussion in high school and collegiate football. *Brain Injury, 20*(1), 33-39.

McCombs, M. (2004). *Setting the agenda: The mass media and public opinion*. Malden, MA: Blackwell Publishing.

McCombs, M. (2005). A look at agenda-setting: Past, present and future. *Journalism Studies, 6*, 543-557.

McCombs, M. E., & Shaw, D. L. (1972). The agenda-setting function of the mass media. *Public Opinion Quarterly, 36*, 176-187.

McCrea, M., Guskiewicz, K. M., Marshall, S. W., Barr, W., Randolph, C., Cantu, R. C., ... Kelly, J. P. (2003, November 19). Acute effects and recovery time following concussion in collegiate football players. *Journal of the American Medical Association, 290*(10), 2556-2563.

McDonald, M. G. (1999). Unnecessary roughness: Gender and racial politics in domestic violence media events. *Sociology of Sports Journal, 16*(2), 111-133.

McDowell, J., & Schaffner, S. (2011). Football, it's a man's game: Insult and gendered discourse in *The Gender Bowl*. *Discourse & Society*, *22*(5), 547-564.

McGannon, K. R., Cunningham, S. M., & Schinke, R. J. (2013). Understanding concussion in a socio-cultural context: A media analysis of a National Hockey League star's concussion. *Psychology of Sport and Exercise*, *14*(6), 891-899.

McGinnis, J. M., & Foege, W. H. (1993, November 10). Actual causes of death in the United States. *Journal of the American Medical Association*, *270*(18), 2207-2212.

McIntosh, W. D., Bazzini, D. G., Smith, S. M., & Wayne, S. M. (1998). Who smokes in Hollywood? Characteristics of smokers in popular films from 1940 to 1989. *Addictive Behaviors*, *23*, 395-398.

McKee, A. C., Cairns, N. J., Dickson, D. W., Folkerth, R. D., Keene, C. D., Litvan, I., … the TBI/CTE Group. (2016). The first NINDS/NIBIB consensus meeting to define neuropathological criteria for the diagnosis of chronic traumatic encephalopathy. *Acta Neuropathologica*, *131*(1), 75-86.

McKee, A. C., Cantu, R. C., Nowinski, C. J., Hedley-Whyte, E. T., Gavett, B. E., Budson, A. E., … Stern, R. A. (2009). Chronic traumatic encephalopathy in athletes: Progressive tauopathy after repetitive head injury. *Journal of Neuropathology & Experimental Neurology*, *68*(7), 709-735.

McKee, A. C., Stein, T. D., Nowinksi, C. J., Stern, R. A., Daneshvar, D. H., Alvarez, V. E., … Cantu, R. C. (2013, January). The spectrum of disease in chronic traumatic encephalopathy. *Brain*, *136*(1), 43-64.

McNamee, M. (2014). Professional football, concussion, and the obligation to protect head injured players. *Sport, Ethics and Philosophy*, *8*(2), 113-115.

Meggyesy, D. (2000). Athletes in big-time college sport. *Society*, *37*(3), 24-28.

Mendez, M. F. (1995). The neuropsychiatric aspects of boxing. *International Journal of Psychiatry in Medicine*, *25*(3), 249-262.

Merz, Z. C., Van Patten, R., & Lace, J. (2017). Current public knowledge pertaining to traumatic brain injury: Influence of demographic factors, social trends, and sport concussion experience on the understanding of traumatic brain injury sequelae. *Archives of Clinical Neuropsychology*, *32*, 155-167.

Messner, M. (1990). When bodies are weapons: Masculinity and violence in sport. *International Review for the Sociology of Sport*, *25*(3), 203-218.

Messner, M. (2012). Reflections on communication and sport: On men and masculinities. *Communication & Sport*, *1*(1/2), 113-124.

Mez, J., Daneshvar, D. H., Klernan, P. T., Abdolmohammadl, B., Alvarez, V. E., Huber, B. R., … McKee, A. C. (2017). Clinicopathological evaluation of chronic traumatic encephalopathy in player of American Football. *Journal of the American Medical Association*, *318*(4), 360-370.

Michaels, D. (2008). *Doubt is their product: How industry's assault on science threatens your health*. New York, NY: Oxford University Press.

Middlehurst-Schwartz, M. (2015, March 16). Chris Borland retiring out of concern for head injuries. *USA Today*. Retrieved July 13, 2018, from https://www.usatoday.com/story/sports/nfl/ 9ers/2015/03/16/chris-borland-retire-san-francisco-49ers-head-injuries-concussion/24882901/

Middlehurst-Schwartz, M. (2016, March 20). Seahawks' Richard Sherman: Roger Goodell "foolish" for ejection proposal. *USA Today*. Retrieved July 14, 2018, from https://www.usatoday.com/story/sports/nfl/seahawks/2016/03/20/richard-sherman-roger-goodell-foolish-ejection-proposal/82050612/

Miller, J. A., & Belson, K. (2013, August 24). N.F.L. said to have pressured ESPN. *New York Times*, D1.

Miller, T. (2014). NFL sex. In T. P. Oates & Z. Furness (Eds.), *The NFL: Critical and cultural perspectives* (pp. 103-118). Philadelphia, PA: Temple University Press.

Mills, R. (1997, July 24). A man of steel crumbles. *St. Petersburg Times*, 1C.

Millspaugh, J. A. (1937). Dementia pugilistica. *United States Naval Medical Bulletin*, *35*(1), 297-303.

Mokdad, A. H., Marks, J. S., Stroup, D. F., & Gerberding, J. L. (2004, March 10). Actual causes of death in the United States. *Journal of the American Medical Association, 291*(10), 1238-1245.

Molotch, H., & Lester, M. (1974). News as purposive behavior: On the strategic use of routine events, accidents, and scandals. *American Sociological Review, 39*(1), 101-112.

Montenigro, P. H., Bernick, C., & Cantu, R. C. (2015). Clinical features of repetitive traumatic brain injury and chronic traumatic encephalopathy. *Brain Pathology, 25*(3), 304-317.

Montenigro, P. H., Sisniega, D. C., & Cantu, R. C. (2016a). Cumulative effects of repeated mild traumatic brain injury and chronic traumatic encephalopathy. In F. S. Zollman (Ed.), *Manual of traumatic brain injury: Assessment and management* (2nd ed.) (pp. 438-446). New York: Springer.

Montenigro, P. H., Sisniega, D. C., & Cantu, R. C. (2016b). Sport-related concussion I: Injury prevention and initial assessment. In F. S. Zollman (Ed.), *Manual of traumatic brain injury: Assessment and management* (2nd ed.) (pp. 65-70). New York: Springer.

Montez de Oca, J. (2013). *Discipline and indulgence: College football, media, and the American way of life during the Cold War*. New Brunswick NJ: Rutgers University Press.

Montez de Oca, J., Meyer, B., & Scholes, J. (2016). Reaching the kids: NFL youth marketing and media. *Popular Communication, 14*(1), 3-11.

Moon, K., & Theodore, N. (2016, May). Football and chronic traumatic encephalopathy: How much evidence actually exists? *World Neurosurgery News, 89*, 720-721.

Moser, A., & Miller, J. J. (2014). Mismanaging concussions in intercollegiate football. *Journal of Physical Education, Recreation & Dance, 85*(2), 38-40.

Moughty, S. (2013, August 22). A note from FRONTLINE: ESPN and "League of Denial." Retrieved February 2, 2018, from https://www.pbs.org/wgbh/frontline/article/a-note-from-frontline-espn-and-league-of-denial/

Murphy, A. (1999, August 30). The boy czar strikes television gold. *Sports Illustrated, 91*(8), 82-83.

Murphy, P., & Waddington, I. (2007). Are elite athletes exploited? *Sport in Society: Cultures, Commerce, Media, Politics, 10*(2), 239-255.

Myers, G. (1989). The pragmatics of politeness in scientific articles. *Applied Linguistics, 10*(1), 1-35.

Myers, G. (2016, October 9). How ten year of Roger Goodell as NFL commissioner has transformed the league and shaped his legacy. *New York Daily News.* http://www.nydailynews.com/sports/football/best-worst-roger-goodell-10-years-nfl-commissioner-article-1.2824168

Nair, Y. (2000). Dead images, live transmissions: Greg Louganis and the construction of AIDS on television. *Discourse, 22*(1), 53-69.

Naiyer, N., Chounthirath, T., & Smith, G. A. (2017). Pediatric cheerleading injuries treated in emergency departments in the United States. *Clinical Pediatrics, 56*(11), 985-992.

National Football League. (2007, August 14). *NFL outlines for players steps taken to address concussions* [Press release]. Retrieved from http://www.nfl.com/news/story/09000d5d8017cc67/article/nfl-outlines-for-players-steps-taken-to-address-concussions

Neale, T. (2009, December 3). NFL institutes new concussion policy. *Medpage Today*. Retrieved September 22, 2017, from https://www.medpagetoday.com/Neurology/HeadTrauma/17302

Nelson, R. R. (1959). The simple economics of basic scientific research. *Journal of Political Economy, 67*(3), 297-306.

Neuman, R. W., Just, M. R., & Crigler, A. N. (1992). *Common knowledge: News and the construction of political meaning*. Chicago: University of Chicago Press.

Newkirk II, V. R. (2017, September 29). Football has always been a battleground in the culture war. *The Atlantic*. Retrieved July 5, 2018, from https://www.theatlantic.com/politics/archive/2017/09/football-is-the-culture-war/541464/

NFL announces Play Smart. Play Safe., A new commitment to improve player health and safety. (2016). Retrieved September 22, 2017, from https://nflcommunications.com/Pages/NFL-Announces-Play-Smart.-Play-Safe.,-a-New-Commitment-to-Improve-Player-Health-and-Safety.aspx

NFL donates $30 million to National Institutes of Health. (2012, September 5). Retrieved September 15, 2017, from http://www.nfl.com/news/story/0ap1000000058447/article/nfl-donates-30-million-to-national-institutes-of-health

Nichols, B. (1991). *Representing reality: Issues and concepts in documentary*. Bloomington, IN: Indiana University Press.

Nichols, E. H., & Smith, H. B. (1906, January 4). The physical aspect of American football. *The Boston Medical and Surgical Journal, 154*, 1-8.

Nierenberg, A. A. (2017). Defensible or not? *Psychiatric Annals, 47*(12), 571-572.

NIH chronic traumatic encephalopathy diagnosis conference. (n.d.). Retrieved September 14, 2017, from https://www.ninds.nih.gov/Current-Research/Focus-Research/Traumatic-Brain-Injury/NIH-Chronic-Traumatic-Encephalopathy

NIH, NFL, and concussion research funding. (2014, February). *The Journal of Nuclear Medicine, 55*(2), 12N.

Nixon II, H. L. (1993). Accepting the risks of pain and injury in sport: Mediated cultural influences on playing hurt. *Sociology of Sport Journal, 10*(2), 183-196.

Noar, S. M., Francis, D. B., Bridges, C., Sontag, J. M., Ribisl, K. M., & Brewer, N. T. (2016). The impact of strengthening cigarette pack warnings: Systematic review of longitudinal observational studies. *Social Science & Medicine, 164*, 118-129.

Nowinski, C. (2007). *Head games: Football's concussion crisis*. East Bridgewater, MA: The Drummond Publishing Group.

Oaklander, M., Park, A., Ducharme, J., & Marty, R. (2018, October 29). 50 most influential people in health care. *Time, 192*(17), pp. 33-41.

Oates, T. P. (2017). *Football and manliness: An unauthorized feminist account of the NFL*. Urbana, IL: University of Illinois Press.

Often misdiagnosed as Alzheimer's disease, chronic traumatic encephalopathy could play a role in veterans' dementia. (2011, May 19). *U.S. Medicine*. Retrieved July 10, 2018, from http://www.usmedicine.com/agencies/department-of-defense-dod/often-misdiagnosed-as-alzheimers-disease-chronic-traumatic-encephalopathy-could-play-a-role-in-veterans-dementia/

Omalu, B. I. (2004). Chronic traumatic encephalopathy and the National Football League. *Journal of Neuropathology & Experimental Neurology, 63*(5), 535.

Omalu, B. (2008). *Play hard, die young: Football dementia, depression, and death*. Lodi, CA: Neo-Forenxis Books.

Omalu, B. (2015, December 7). Don't let kids play football. *New York Times*, p. A23.

Omalu, B. I., DeKosky, S. T., Hamilton, R. L., Minster, R. L., Kamboh, M. I., Shakir, A. M., & Wecht, C. H. (2006). Chronic traumatic encephalopathy in a National Football League player: Part II. *Neurosurgery, 59*(5), 1086-1092.

Omalu, B. I., DeKosky, S. T., Minster, R. L., Kamboh, M. I., Hamilton, R. L., & Wecht, C. H. (2005). Chronic traumatic encephalopathy in a National Football League player. *Neurosurgery, 57*(1), 128-134.

Omalu, B. I., Fitzsimmons, R. P., Hammers, J., & Bailes, J. (2010). Chronic traumatic encephalopathy in a professional American wrestler. *Journal of Forensic Nursing, 6*, 130-136.

Omalu, B., Hammers, J. L., Bailes, J., Hamilton, R. L., Kamboh, M. I., Webster, G., & Fitzsimmons, R. P. (2011). Chronic traumatic encephalopathy in an Iraqi war veteran with posttraumatic stress disorder who committed suicide. *Neurosurgical Focus, 31*(5), 1-12.

Omalu, B., Small, G. W., Bailes, J., Ercoli, L. M., Merrill, D. A., Wong, K., ... Barrio, J. R. (2018, February). Postmortem autopsy-confirmation of antemortem [F-18] FDDNP-PET scans in a football player with chronic traumatic encephalopathy. *Neurosurgery, 82*(2), 237-246.

O'Neill, D., & Harcup, T. (2009). News values and selectivity. In K. Wahl-Jorgensen & T. Hanitzsch (Eds.), *The handbook of journalism studies*, (pp. 161-174). New York: Routledge.

O'Phelan, K. (2016). Traumatic brain injury: Definitions and nomenclature. In F. S. Zollman (Ed.), *Manual of traumatic brain injury: Assessment and management* (2nd ed.) (pp. 3-9). New York: Springer.

Oreskes, N., & Conway, E. (2010). *Merchants of doubt: How a handful of scientists obscured the truth on issues from tobacco smoke to global warming*. New York, NY: Bloomsbury Press.

Oriard, M. (1993). *Reading football: How the popular press created an American spectacle*. Chapel Hill, NC: The University of North Carolina Press.

Oriard, M. (2007). *Brand NFL: Making and selling America's favorite sport*. Chapel Hill, NC: University of North Carolina Press.

Oriard, M. (2014a). Chronicle of a (football) death foretold: The imminent demise of a national pastime? *The International Journal of the History of Sport*, *31*(1-2), 120-133.

Oriard, M. (2014b). Foreword: Football as mediated spectacle. In T. P. Oates & Z. Furness (Eds.), *The NFL: Critical and cultural perspectives* (pp. vii-x). Philadelphia, PA: Temple University Press.

Ortiz, R. (2016, February 10). Concussions—Happens in other sports than football. *Los Angeles Times*. Retrieved July 13, 2018, from http://highschool.latimes.com/bonita-high-school/concussions-happens-in-other-sports-than-football/

Osborn, J. E. (1986). The AIDS epidemic: An overview of the science. *Issues in Science and Technology*, *2*, 40-55.

Otero, E. (2015, June 25). Football causes most concussions? Think again. *News Leader*. Retrieved July 13, 2018, from https://www.newsleader.com/story/sports/2015/06/25/concussions-soccer-football-wrestling/29268651/

Páez, D., Echebarria, A., Valencia, J., Romo, I., San Juan, C., & Vergara, A. (1991). AIDS social representations: Contents and processes. *Journal of Community and Applied SocialPsychology*, *1*, 89-104.

Paolini, M. (2019). NFL takes a page from the Big Tobacco playbook: Assumption of risk in the CTE crisis. *Emory Law Journal*, *68*(3), 607-642.

Pappas, N. T., McKenry, P. C., & Catlett, B. S. (2004). Athlete aggression on the rink and off the ice: Athlete violence and aggression in hockey and interpersonal relationships. *Men and Masculinities*, *6*(3), 291-312.

Parker, H. L. (1934). Traumatic encephalopathy ("punch drunk") of professional pugilists. *The Journal of Neurology and Psychopathology*, *15*(57), 20-28.

Parrott, R. (1996). Advocate or adversary? The self-reflexive role of media messages for health. *Critical Studies in Mass Communication*, *13*, 266-278.

Pasquarelli, L. (1997, July 25). Humbled hero; Webster fights to overcome despair. *The Atlanta Journal-Constitution*, p. 4E.

Patricios, J. S., & Kemp, S. (2014). Chronic traumatic encephalopathy: Rugby's call for clarity, data and leadership in the concussion debate. *British Journal of Sports Medicine*, *48*(2), 76-79.

Patriotta, G., & Gruber, D. A. (2015). Newsmaking and sensemaking: Navigating temporal transitions between planned and unexpected events. *Organization Science*, *26*(6), 1574-1592.

Patton, C. (1990). *Inventing AIDS*. New York, NY: Routledge.

Payne, J. G., & Mercuri, K. A. (1993). Crisis in communication: Coverage of Magic Johnson's AIDS disclosure. In S. C. Raztan (Ed.), *AIDS: Effective health communication for the 90s* (pp. 151-172). Boston: Taylor & Francis.

Pellman, E. J., & Viano, D. C. (2006, October). Concussions in professional football. *Neurosurgical Focus*, *21*(4), 1-10.

Pellman, E. J., Viano, D. C., Casson, I. R., Arfken, C., & Feuer, H. (2005, January). Concussion in professional football: Players returning to the same game—part 7. *Neurosurgery*, *56*(1), 79-90.

Pellman, E. J., Viano, D. C., Casson, I. R., Tucker, A. M., Waeckerle, J. F., Powell, J. W., & Feuer, H. (2004, October). Concussion in professional football: Repeat injuries—part 4. *Neurosurgery, 55*(4), 860-876.

Pellman, E. J., Viano, D. C., Tucker, A. M., Casson, I. R., & Waeckerle, J. F. (2003, October). Concussion in professional football: Reconstruction of game impacts and injuries. *Neurosurgery, 53*(4), 799-814.

Pennington, B. (2004, May 18). Sports turnaround: The team doctors now pay the team. *New York Times*. Retrieved July 3, 2018, from https://www.nytimes.com/2004/05/18/sports/sports-medicine-sports-turnaround-the-team-doctors-now-pay-the-team.html

Pennington, B. (2017, November 23). As concussion worries rise, girls' lacrosse turns to headgear. *New York Times.* Retrieved July 13, 2018, from https://www.nytimes.com/2017/11/23/sports/girls-lacrosse-concussions-headgear.html

Perrine, K., Helcer, J., Tsiouris, A. J., Pisapia, D. J., & Stieg, P. (2017, June). The current status of research on chronic traumatic encephalopathy. *World Neurosurgery, 102,* 533-544.

Peter, J. (2017, January 31). NFL legend Earl Campbell still hits hard, compares current NFL to wrestling. *USA Today.* Retrieved July 14, 2018, from https://www.usatoday.com/story/sports/nfl/super/2017/01/31/earl-campbell-super-bowl-li-51-houston-oilers-texas-running-back-pain-gain-pro-football-hall-of-fame/97258738/

Phillips, E. B. (1976). Novelty without change. *Journal of Communication, 26*(4), 87-92.

Pierce, J. P., & Gilpin, E. A. (2001, June). News media coverage of smoking and health is associated with changes in population rates of smoking cessation but not initiation. *Tobacco Control, 10*(2), 145-153.

Pierson, D. (2002, September 25). It was game that claimed ex-Steeler. *Chicago Tribune.* Retrieved August 21, 2017, from http://articles.chicagotribune.com/2002-09-25/news/0209250294_1_brain-damage-mike-webster-garrett-webster

Posthuma, R. A., Flores, G. L., Barlow, M. A., & Dworkin, J. B. (2018). Social signaling and interorganizational relationships: Lessons learned from the professional sports industry. *Business Horizons, 61*(4), 521-531.

Pöttker, H. (2003). News and its communicative quality: The inverted pyramid—when and why did it appear? *Journalism Studies, 4*(4), 501-511.

Powell, M. (2017, February 4). Tagliabue's flawed legacy. *New York Times*, D1.

Practice parameter: The management of concussion in sports (summary statement). (1997, March 1). *Neurology, 48*, 581-585.

Proctor, R. N., & Schiebinger, L. (2008). *Agnotology: The making & unmaking of ignorance.* Stanford, CA: Stanford University Press.

Rabinovici, G. D. (2017, July 25). Advances and gaps in understanding chronic traumatic encephalopathy: From pugilists to American football players. *Journal of the American Medical Association, 318*(4), 338-340.

Ramsey, T. (2017, December 21). Alternative sports gaining popularity among youth. *WS Chronicle.* Retrieved July 13, 2018, from http://www.wschronicle.com/2017/12/alternative-sports-gaining-popularity-among-youth/

Randolph, C. (2011, January/February). Baseline neuropsychological testing in managing sport-related concussion: Does it modify risk? *Current Sports Medicine Reports, 10*(1), 21-26.

Randolph, C. (2014, January/February). Is chronic traumatic encephalopathy a real disease? *Current Sports Medicine Reports, 13*(1), 33-37.

Randolph, C. (2018, August). Chronic traumatic encephalopathy is not a real disease. *Archives of Clinical Neuropsychology, 33*(5), 644-648.

Real, M. R. (1975). Super Bowl: Mythic spectacle. *Journal of Communication, 25*(1), 31-43.

Reardon, K. K., & Richardson, J. L. (1991). The important role of mass media in the diffusion of accurate information about AIDS. *Journal of Homosexuality, 21*(1-2), 63-76. doi: 10.1300/J082v21no1_06

Reid, M. W., & Velez, C. S. (2015). Discriminating military and civilian traumatic brain injuries. *Molecular and Cellular Neuroscience, 66*(Part B), 123-128.

Reider, B. (2013). Headlines. *The American Journal of Sports Medicine, 41*(12), 2739-2741.

Reynolds, B. B., Patrie, J., Henry, E. J., Goodkin, H. P., Broshek, D. K., Wintermark, M., & Druzgal, J. (2016). Quantifying head impacts in collegiate lacrosse. *The American Journal of Sports Medicine, 44*(11), 2947-2956.

Ricketson, M. (2016). When slow news is good news. *Journalism Practice, 10*(4), 507-520.

Riffe, D., Lacy, S., & Fico, F. G. (2005). *Analyzing media messages: Using quantitative content analysis in research* (2nd ed.). Rahway, NJ: Lawrence Erlbaum Associates.

Robbins, B. (1997). Head fake: Mentorship and mobility in *Hoop Dreams. Social Text, 50*, 111-120.

Roberts, A. H. (1969). *Brain damage in boxers: A study of the prevalence of traumatic encephalopathy among ex-professional boxers*. London: Pitman Medical and Scientific Publishing Co.

Roberts, G. W., Allsop, D., & Bruton, C. (1990). The occult aftermath of boxing. *Journal of Neurology, Neurosurgery, and Psychiatry, 53*(5), 373-378.

Roberts, G. W., Whitwell, H. L., Acland, P. R., & Bruton, C. J. (1990, April). Dementia in a punch-drunk wife. *The Lancet, 335*(8694), 918-919.

Rodgers, K. (2014). "I was a gladiator": Pain, injury, and masculinity in the NFL. In T. P. Oates & Z. Furness (Eds.), *The NFL: Critical and cultural perspectives* (pp. 142-159). Philadelphia, PA: Temple University Press.

Rodrigues, J. (2009, March 31). When smoking was cool, cheap, legal and socially acceptable. *The Guardian*. Retrieved from https://www.theguardian.com/lifeandstyle/2009/apr/01/tobacco-industry-marketing

Rogers, E. M., Dearing, J. W., & Chang, S. (1991). AIDS in the 1980s: The agenda-setting process for a public issue. *Journalism Monographs*, 126.

Rollow, C. (1989, August 6). Bradshaw makes big play at Hall of Fame. *Chicago Tribune*. Retrieved August 21, 2017, from http://articles.chicagotribune.com/1989-08-06/sports/8901030369_1_terry-bradshaw-steeler-fense

Rosenberg, H. (1985, January 11). Football glory doesn't always hurt so good. *Los Angeles Times*. Retrieved December 22, 2017, from http://articles.latimes.com/1985-01-11/entertainment/ca-8569_1_football-glory

Roth, M. (2013, May 13). Scientists hunt for ways to untangle damage of CTE. *Pittsburgh Post-Gazette*, p. A-1.

Sabo, D. (2009). Sports injury, the pain principle, and the promise of reform. *Journal of Intercollegiate Sports, 2*(1), 145-152.

Sabo, D., & Gordon, D. F. (1995). Rethinking men's health and illness. In D. Sabo & D. F. Gordon (Eds.), *Men's health and illness: Gender, power, and the body* (pp. 1-21). Thousand Oaks, CA: Sage.

Sabo, D., & Jansen, S. C. (1992). Images of men in sport media: The social reproduction of gender order. In S. Craig (Ed.), *Men, masculinity, and the media* (pp. 169-185). Newbury Park, CA: Sage.

Sabo, D. F., & Panepinto, J. (1990). Football ritual and the social reproduction of masculinity. In M. A. Messner & D. F. Sabo (Eds.), *Sport, men, and the gender order: Critical feminist perspectives* (pp. 115-126). Champaign, IL: Human Kinetics.

Sacks, V. (1996). Women and AIDS: An analysis of media misrepresentations. *Social Science & Medicine, 42*(1), 59-73.

Saffary, R., Chin, L. S., & Cantu, R. C. (2012). From concussion to chronic traumatic encephalopathy. *Journal of Clinical Sport Psychology, 6*, 351-362.

Sage, G. H. (1998). *Power and ideology in American sport: A critical perspective* (2nd ed.). Champaign, IL: Human Kinetics.

Salamon, M. (2015, December 10). Concussions are biggest health risk to cheerleaders. Retrieved July 12, 2018, from https://consumer.healthday.com/cognitive-health-information-26/concussions-news-733/concussions-are-biggest-health-risk-to-cheerleaders-706029.html

Salleh, A. (2001). Science in the media: The good, the bad and the ugly. *Australian Science Teachers' Journal, 47*(4), 28-37.
Samuel, E. (2016, March 21). Sherman levels Rogers: Says commish is "just a suit." *New York Daily News*, p. 50.
Sandman, P. M. (1994). Mass media and environmental risk: Seven principles. *Risk: Health, Safety & Environment, 5*(3), 251-260.
Sanderson, J., Weathers, M., Grevious, A., Tehan, M., & Warren, S. (2016). A hero or sissy? Exploring media framing of NFL quarterbacks injury decisions. *Communication & Sport, 4*(1), 3-22.
Schad, T. (2017, October 31). Myles Garrett on why he self-reported concussions: "I can't play around with my brain." *USA Today*. https://www.usatoday.com/story/sports/nfl/browns/2017/10/31/myles-garrett-concussion-self-reported-cleveland-browns/819234001/
Schatz, P., & Moser, R. S. (2011). Current issues in pediatric sports concussion. *The Clinical Neuropsychologist, 25*(6), 1042-1057.
Scheufele, D. A. (1999). Framing as a theory of media effects. *Journal of Communication, 49*(1), 103-122.
Scheufele, D. A., & Tewksbury, D. (2007). Framing, agenda setting, and priming: The evolution of three media effects models. *Journal of Communication, 57*(1), 9-20.
Schiavo, R. (2007). *Health communication: From theory to practice.* San Francisco, CA: Jossey Bass.
Schneider, J., & Eitzen, D. S. (2010). The structure of sport and participant violence. In R. E. Washington & D. Karen (Eds.), *Sport, power, and society: Institutions and practices* (pp. 409-421). New York: Westview Press.
Schudson, M. (1986). Deadlines, datelines, and history. In R. K. Manoff & M. Schudson (Eds.), *Reading the news: A pantheon guide to popular culture* (pp. 79-108). New York: Pantheon Books.
Schudson, M. (1989). The sociology of news production. *Media, Culture, & Society, 11*(3), 263-282.
Schwarz, A. (2007a, January 18). Expert ties ex-player's suicide to brain damage from football. *New York Times*, p. A1.
Schwarz, A. (2007b, June 20). Player silence on concussions may block N.F.L. guidelines. *New York Times*, p. A1.
Schwarz, A. (2009, December 3). New N.F.L. rule on concussions benches injuries. *New York Times*, pp. A1, A3.
Schwarz, A. (2011, May 3). Duerson's brain trauma diagnosed. *New York Times*, p. B11.
Schwarz, A. (2016, July 27). N.F.L.-backed youth program says it reduced concussions. The data disagrees. *New York Times*. Retrieved July 11, 2018, from http://www.nytimes.com/2016/07/28/sports/football/nfl-concussions-youth-program-heads-up-football.html?partner=bloomberg
Schwarz, A., Bogdanich, W., & Williams, J. (2016, March 24). N.F.L.'s flawed concussion research and ties to tobacco industry. *New York Times*. Retrieved June 11, 2018, from https://www.nytimes.com/2016/03/25/sports/football/nfl-concussion-research-tobacco.html?_r=0
Scott, D. (2017). Boxing: From male vocation to neurotic masculinity. *Sport in History, 37*(4), 469-482.
Scott, R., Scott, G., Wolthoff, D., Shuman, L., & Cantillon, E. (Producers), Landesman, P. (Director). (2015). *Concussion*. [Motion Picture]. United States: Columbia Pictures.
Seifert, K. (2016a, July 21). NFL medical adviser Elliot Pellman retiring; move prompted by Roger Goodell. Retrieved September 21, 2017, from http://www.espn.com/nfl/story/_/id/17113610/controversial-nfl-medical-adviser-elliot-pellman-retiring
Seifert, K. (2016b, August 8). Ten ways the NFL has changed under Roger Goodell. *ESPN*. Retrieved from http://tv5.espn.com/blog/nflnation/post/_/id/208754/ten-ways-the-nfl-has-changed-under-roger-goodell
Sexton, P. (1969). *The feminized male*. New York: Random House.

Shapiro, I. (2010). Evaluating journalism. *Journalism Practice*, *4*(2), 143-162.
Sharp, D. J., & Jenkins, P. O. (2015). Concussion is confusing us all. *Practical Neurology*, *15*(3), 172-186.
Shaw, G. (2013, October 17). What did the NFL know and when and what could neurology have done? *Neurology Today*, *13*(20), 1, 16-18.
Shell, A. (2017, September 5). Why families stretch their budgets for high-priced youth sports. *USA Today*. Retrieved July 13, 2018, from https://www.usatoday.com/story/money/2017/09/05/why-families-stretch-their-budgets-high-priced-youth-sports/571945001/
Sidibé, M. (2018). Foreword. *UNAIDS data 2018*. Retrieved December 17, 2018, from http://www.unaids.org/sites/default/files/media_asset/unaids-data-2018_en.pdf
Siegler, J. E., & Wesley, S. F. (2016, October 4). Right brain: *Concussion* (film) review and historical context. *Neurology*, *87*, e155-e158.
Sigal, L. V. (1986). Sources make the news. In R. K. Manoff & M. Schudson (Eds.), *Reading the news: A pantheon guide to popular culture* (pp. 9-37). New York: Pantheon Books.
Signorielli, N. (1990). Television and health: Images and impact. In C. Atkin & L. Wallack (Eds.), *Mass communication and public health* (pp. 96-113). New Delhi, India: Sage.
Signorielli, N. (1998). Health images on television. In L. D. Jackson (Ed.), *Health communication research: A guide to developments and directions* (pp. 163-179). Westport, CT: Greenwood.
Silverberg, N. D., Lange, R. T., & Iverson, G. L. (2016). Concussion and mild traumatic brain injury: Definitions, distinctions, and diagnostic criteria. In F. S. Zollman (Ed.), *Manual of traumatic brain injury: Assessment and management* (2nd ed.), (pp. 43-49). New York: Springer. 2016.
Slater, M. D., Long, M., Bettinghaus, E. P., & Reineke, J. B. (2008). News coverage of cancer in the United States: A national sample of newspapers, television, and magazines. *Journal of Health Communication*, *13*(6), 523-537. doi: 10.1080/10810730802279571
Smith, D. H., & Stewart, W. (2016, June). Tackling concussion, beyond Hollywood. *The Lancet Neurology*, *15*(7), 662-663.
Smith, R. K. (2013). Solving the concussion problem and saving professional football. *Thomas Jefferson Law Review*, *35*(2), 127-191.
Solomon, G. (2018). Chronic traumatic encephalopathy in sports: A historical and narrative review. *Developmental Neuropsychology*, *43*(4), 279-311.
Solomon, G. S., & Sills, A. (2014). Chronic traumatic encephalopathy and the availability cascade. *The Physician and Sportsmedicine*, *42*(3), 26-31.
Sontag, S. (1988). *AIDS and its metaphors*. New York, NY: Farrar, Straus, and Giroux.
Stade, G. (1966). Game theory. *The Columbia University Forum*, *9*(4), 40-42.
Starkey, J. P. (2013, March). NFL rule changes: The internet responds to Roger Goodell. *SB Nation*. Retrieved July 14, 2018, from https://www.sbnation.com/nfl/2013/3/20/4128546/nfl-rule-changes-roger-goodell
Stein, T. D., Alvarez, V. E., & McKee, A. C. (2015, October). Concussion in chronic traumatic encephalopathy. *Current Pain and Headache Reports*, *19*(10), 1-6.
Stern, R. A., Riley, D. O., Daneshvar, D. H., Nowinski, C. J., Cantu, R. C., & McKee, A. C. (2011, October). Long-term consequences of repetitive brain trauma: Chronic traumatic encephalopathy. *Physical Medicine and Rehabilitation*, *3*(10, Suppl. 2), S460-467.
Strauss, A., & Corbin, J. (1990). *Basics of qualitative research: Grounded theory procedures and techniques*. Newbury Park, CA: Sage.
Strup, J. (2006, July 1). The brothers Fainaru. Retrieved June 7, 2018, from http://www.editorandpublisher.com/news/the-brothers-fainaru/
Swain, K. A. (2005). Approaching the quarter-century mark: AIDS coverage and research decline as infection spreads. *Critical Studies in Media Communication*, *22*(3), 258-262. doi: 10.1080/07393180500206073

Tagilabue, P. (2003, October). Tackling concussions in sports. *Neurosurgery, 53*(4), 796.

Talosig-Garcia, M., & Davis, S. W. (2005). Information-seeking, behavior of minority breast cancer patients: An exploratory study. *Journal of Health Communication, 10*, 53-64.

Tannenbaum, P. H. (1953). The effect of headlines on the interpretation of news stories. *Journalism Quarterly, 30*(2), 189-197.

Tanner, L. (2016, August 23). Fists not football: Brain injuries seen in domestic assaults. *Associated Press*. Retrieved June 22, 2018, from http://www.foxnews.com/health/2016/08/23/fists-not-football-brain-injuries-seen-in-domestic-assaults.html

Tanveer, S., Zecavati, N., Delasobera, E. B., & Oyegbile, T. O. (2017, May). Gender differences in concussion and postinjury cognitive findings in an older and younger pediatric population. *Pediatric Neurology, 70*, 44-49.

Tate, C. (2000). *Cigarette wars: The triumph of the "little white slaver."* New York, NY: Oxford University Press.

Tator, C. H. (2014). Chronic traumatic encephalopathy: How serious a sports problem is it? *British Journal of Sports Medicine, 48*, 81-83.

TBI: Get the facts. (n.d.). *Center for Disease Control and Prevention*. Retrieved September 5, 2017, from https://www.cdc.gov/traumaticbraininjury/get_the_facts.html

Teasdale, G., & Jennett, B. (1974, July 13). Assessment of coma and impaired consciousness: A practical scale. *The Lancet, 304*(7872), 81-84.

Teasdale, G., Maas, A., Lecky, F., Manley, G., Stocchetti, N., & Murray, G. (2014, August). The Glasgow Coma Scale at 40 years: Standing the test of time. *Lancet Neurology, 13*, 844-855.

Teitelbaum, M. (2010). *Sports in America, 1980-1989* (2nd ed.). New York: Chelsea House.

Tobacco Industry Research Committee. (1954, January). A frank statement to cigarette smokers. *The Tobacco Leaf*. Retrieved November 17, 2017, from https://www.industrydocumentslibrary.ucsf.edu/tobacco/docs/#id=ltln0082

Tobacco Master Settlement agreement summary. (2001). Retrieved November 11, 2017, from http://caag.state.ca.us/tobacco/resources/msasumm.htm

Top-US-grossing sports documentaries. (2015). *IMDb.com*. Retrieved December 15, 2015, from http://www.imdb.com/search/title?genres=sport&sort=boxoffice_gross_us&title_type=documentary.

Travis, C., & Holm, P. (2017). Lessons for the Anthropocene from the recent past: Tobacco use, HIV/AIDS, and social transformation. *Global and Planetary Change, 156*, 167-175.

Tuchman, G. (1972). Objectivity as strategic ritual: An examination of newsmen's notions of objectivity. *American Journal of Sociology, 77*(4), 660-679.

Tuchman, G. (1976). Telling stories. *Journal of Communication, 26*(4), 93-97.

Turoe, J., & Coe, L. (1985). Curing television ills: The portrayal of health care. *Journal of Communication, 35*, 36-51.

United States v. Philip Morris et al. (2004). Civil Action No. 99-2496 (GK).

Unterharnscheidt, F., & Taylor-Unterharnscheidt, J. (2003). *Boxing medical aspects*. Amsterdam: Academic Press.

van Dijk, T. A. (1988). *News as discourse*. Hillsdale, NJ: Lawrence Erlbaum Associates.

van Dijk, T. A. (1995). Power and the news media. In D. Paletz (Ed.), *Political communication in action: States, institutions, movements, audiences* (pp. 9-36). Cresskill, NJ: Hampton Press.

van Dijk, T. A. (2009). News, discourse, and ideology. In K. Wahl-Jorgensen & T. Hanitzsch (Eds.), *The handbook of journalism studies*, (pp. 191-204). New York: Routledge.

Vasterman, P. (Ed.). (2018). *From media hype to Twitter storm: News explosions and their impact on issues, crises and public opinion*. Amsterdam: Amsterdam University Press.

Ventresca, M. (2018). The curious case of CTE: Mediating materialities of traumatic brain injury. *Communication & Sport*. https://doi.org/10.1177/2167479518761636

Vescey, G. (1994, December 18). Seeking enlightenment at—where else?—the Y. *New York Times*, p. 5.

Viswanath, K., & Emmons, K. M. (2006). Message effects and social determinants of health: Its application to cancer disparity. *Journal of Communication, 56*, 238-264.

Vogan, T. (2013). NFL Films and the art of selling football. *Popular Communication, 11*(4), 274-288.

Vogan, T. (2014). *Keeper of the flames: NFL Films and the rise of sports media*. Champaign, IL: University of Illinois Press.

Volin, B. (2016, July 9). Why all NFL contracts aren't fully guaranteed. *Boston Globe*. Retrieved July 13, 2018, from https://www.bostonglobe.com/sports/patriots/2016/07/09/why-all-nfl-contracts-aren-fully-guaranteed/99WBMntCztfDjYr8et12qJ/story.html

Vreeman, R. C., & Carroll, A. E. (2007, December). Medical myths. *British Medical Journal, 335*(7633), 1288-1289.

Vrentas, J. (2017, May 31). The quest for a better football helmet. *Sports Illustrated*. Retrieved December 19, 2017, from https://www.si.com/mmqb/2017/05/31/nfl-quest-better-football-helmet

Wachs, F. L., & Dworkin, S. L. (1997). "There's no such thing as a gay hero": Sexual identity and media framing of HIV-positive athletes. *Journal of Sport & Social Issues, 21*(4), 327-347.

Wallace, J., Covassin, T., Nogle, S., Gould, D., & Kovan, J. (2017). Knowledge of concussion and reporting behaviors in high school athletes with or without access to an athletic trainer. *Journal of Athletic Training, 52*(3), 228-235.

Wallenfeldt, E. C. (1994). *The six-minute fraternity: The rise and fall of NCAA tournament boxing, 1932-1960*. Westport, CT: Praeger Publishers.

Walsh-Childers, K. (2017). *Mass media and health: Examining media impact on individuals and the health environment*. New York, NY: Routledge.

Wander, N., & Malone, R. E. (2006). Making big tobacco give in: You lose, they win. *American Journal of Public Health, 96*(11), 2048-2054.

Washington, R. E., & Karen, D. (Eds.). (2010). *Sport, power, and society: Institutions and practices*. Boulder, CO: Westview Press.

Waterhouse-Watson, D. (2013). *Athletes, sexual assault, and "trials by media": Narrative immunity*. New York: Routledge.

Watney, S. (1987). People's perceptions of the risk of AIDS and the role of the mass media. *Health Education Journal, 46*(2), 1-3.

Watney, S. (1989). *Policing desire: Pornography, AIDS, and the media*. Minneapolis, MN: University of Minnesota Press.

Weaver, D. H. (2007). Thoughts on agenda setting, framing, and priming. *Journal of Communication, 57*(1), 142-147.

Weeks, J. (1985). *Sexuality and its discontents: Meanings, myths, and modern sexualities*. New York, NY: Routledge.

Weeks, J. (1989). *AIDS: Social representation, social practices*. Lewes, England: Falmer Press.

Welch, M. (1997). Violence against women by professional football players: A gender analysis of hypermasculinity, positional status, narcissism, and entitlement. *Journal of Sport & Social Issues, 21*(4), 392-411.

Wheelwright, J. (2016). Ahead of the hit. *Discover*, 18-20.

Whiteside, E., & Hardin, M. (2011). Women (not) watching women: Leisure time, television, and implications for televised coverage of women's sports. *Communication, Culture, & Critique*, 4(2), 122-143.

Wilbur, D., & Myers, D. (2016). The NFL and its concussion crisis: Adapting the contingency theory to examine shifts in publics' stances. *Journal of US-China Public Administration, 13*(3), 181-188.

Wilson, D. (2005, March 30). Medical adviser for baseball lists exaggerated credentials. *New York Times*. Retrieved September 22, 2017, from http://www.nytimes.com/2005/

03/30/sports/baseball/medical-adviser-for-baseball-lists-exaggerated-credentials.html?mcubz=0
Wipfli, H., & Samet, J. M. (2016). One hundred years in the making: The global tobacco epidemic. *Annual Review of Public Health, 37,* 149-166.
Wojtys, E. M. (2016). Concussion dilemma. *Sports Health, 8*(1), 17-18.
Wolfson, I. N. (1938, March). Psychiatric aspect of head injuries. *Psychiatric Quarterly, 12*(1), 137-175.
Wood, R. (2016, July 14). Aaron Rodgers opens up about concussions. *USA Today.* Retrieved July 13, 2018, from https://www.packersnews.com/story/sports/nfl/packers/2016/07/14/aaron-rodgers-opens-up-concussions/87076682/
Wortzel, H. S. (2014). Chronic traumatic encephalopathy: Should we be worried? *Psychiatric Times, 31*(4), 12.
Yanovitzsky, I. (2002). Effects of news coverage on policy attention and actions: A closer look at the media-policy connection. *Communication Research, 29,* 422-451.
Yanovitzsky, I., & Bennett, C. (1999). Media attention, institutional response, and health behavior change: The case of drunk driving, 1978-1996. *Communication Research, 26,* 429-453.
Yarnell, P. R., & Lynch, S. (1970, April 25). Retrograde memory immediately after concussion. *The Lancet, 295*(7652), 863-864.
Young, K., White, P., & McTeer, W. (1994). Body talk: Male athletes reflect on sport, injury, and pain. *Sociology of Sport Journal, 11,* 175-194.
Zasler, N. D. (2015). Sports concussion headache. *Brain Injury, 29*(2), 207-220.
Zelizer, B. (2008). Why memory's work on journalism does not reflect journalism's work on memory. *Memory Studies, 1*(1), 79-87.
Zelizer, B., Park, D., & Gudelunas, D. (2002). How bias shapes the news: Challenging *The New York Times'* status as a newspaper of record on the Middle East. *Journalism, 3*(3), 283-307.
Zezima, K. (2014, May 29). How Teddy Roosevelt helped save football. *Washington Post*. Retrieved September 5, 2017, from https://www.washingtonpost.com/news/the-fix/wp/2014/05/29/teddy-roosevelt-helped-save-football-with-a-white-house-meeting-in-1905/?utm_term=.467f55436148

Index

About the Authors

Travis R. Bell (Ph.D., University of South Florida) is an assistant professor of digital and sports media in the Zimmerman School of Advertising & Mass Communications at the University of South Florida. His research interests include sports communication, media framing, race and media, and documentary filmmaking. A former sports broadcast journalist, he is an author on more than a dozen publications about media and film, and producer of five documentary films.

Janelle Applequist (Ph.D., Pennsylvania State University) is an assistant professor of advertising in the Zimmerman School of Advertising & Mass Communications at the University of South Florida. Her research interests include qualitative research methods, pharmaceutical advertising, advertising, health communication, and direct-to-patient recruitment methods for clinical trials. She is the author of *Broadcast Pharmaceutical Advertising in the United States: Primetime Pill Pushers* (2016).

Christian Dotson-Pierson (Ph.D., Howard University) is a speech instructor at the University of South Carolina. An avid sports fan, her professional experiences includes two years working with the Atlanta Braves and in several capacities at KABC-TV. Her research interests include media studies, sports communication, and issues of race and gender.